ANOTHER DIMENSION TO CLINICAL SKILLS EDUCATION

USING VIRTUAL HUMANS, SIMULATION, AND ACTING CONCEPTS TO ENHANCE STANDARDIZED PATIENT TRAINING

Dr. Joel Palathinkal

PRINTED IN THE UNITED STATES OF AMERICA

Visit our website at www.dreemvest.com

The Library of Congress has cataloged the paperback edition as follows:

Palathinkal, Joel John

Another Dimension to Clinical Skills Education

Joel Palathinkal. – 1st ed

1.Medical-Education and Training

2.Medical-Health Policy

3 Medical-Physician and Patient

ISBN-10: 0985381604
ISBN-13: 978-0-9853816-0-8

Book Cover design and Interior Design by Glen M. Edelstein

TABLE OF CONTENTS

LIST OF FIGURES

LIST OF TABLES

This book is dedicated to my family, friends, mentors, and the innovative leaders who continue to push technology and creativity in design; despite the discouragement given from skeptics. Scientific advancements, when not discovered by mistake, were created through perseverance and faith. When not solely through perseverance, individuals of the past who have stood through adversity to take a stand for what they believe in have motivated the individuals of present day. In the future, we should continue making these bold strides; as each influential milestone will be a stepping stone for mankind, progress, and peace on earth.

"Take your budding idea, revolutionize it to change the world, and then unleash it to the masses."

Dr. Joel Palathinkal

ACKNOWLEDGMENTS

It is impossible to quantify the actual time and effort it takes to raise a child. Not only does it take two loving parents, but it truly takes a village to raise a child. My parents (John and Elsamma Palathinkal) utilized the values and beliefs that were instilled in them to constantly nurture a strong marriage; which later fortunately became the backbone of a strong family unit. My brother Joby constantly kept me laughing. These aspects later reflected the way I was raised; and allowed me to be grateful for all the blessings that I was given. I am forever gracious for having a supportive family.

Bill Clinton once said that his major successes were significantly relevant to the friendships that were developed in his lifetime. In addition, Woody Allen said that "80% of success is showing up on time". I completely agree with both of these strong points for if I didn't have the strong professional, personal, and educational support groups, along with the perfectly timed instances of opportunities, I would not be where I am today.

A special and important thanks goes to all that were involved and supportive in the development of this book.

FOREWORD AUTHOR BIOGRAPHY

Dr. Richard M. Satava, MD FACS

I asked Dr. Richard Satava to be my mentor as I was highly inspired by the groundbreaking lectures that he would give at several medical simulation conferences. I reached out to him later to be an advisor for my PhD committee and he was happy to be involved despite his busy schedule. Then after graduating with my PhD, he generously accepted to write the FOREWORD for my first book. Among being one of the first attempted surgeons in space and a pioneer of the first surgical robot that we now know as the Da Vinci Surgical System, below are some of Dr. Satava's honored achievements (Flanagan, 2008).

"Richard Satava, MD, FACS, is Professor of Surgery at the University of Washington Medical Center, and Senior Science Advisor at the US Army Medical Research and Materiel Command in Ft. Detrick, MD. Prior positions include Professor of Surgery at Yale University and a military appointment as Professor of Surgery (USUHS) in the Army Medical Corps assigned to General Surgery at Walter Reed Army Medical Center and Program Manager of Advanced Biomedical Technology at the Defense Advanced Research Projects Agency (DARPA).

His undergraduate training was at Johns Hopkins University, medical school at Hahnemann University of Philadelphia, internship at the Cleveland Clinic, surgical residency at the Mayo Clinic, and a fellowship with a Master of Surgical Research at Mayo Clinic.

He has served on the White House Office of Science and Technology Policy (OSTP) Committee on Health, Food and Safety. He is currently a member of the Emerging Technologies and Resident Education, and Informatics committees of the American College of Surgeons (ACS), is past president of the

Society of American Gastrointestinal Endoscopic Surgeons (SAGES), past president of the Society of Laparoendoscopic Surgeons (SLS), and is on the Board of Governors of the National Board of Medical Examiners (NBME) as well as on a number of surgical societies. He is on the editorial board of numerous surgical and scientific journals, and active in numerous surgical and engineering societies.

He has been continuously active in surgical education and surgical research, with more than 200 publications and book chapters in diverse areas of advanced surgical technology, including Surgery in the Space Environment, Video and 3-D imaging, Telepresence Surgery, Virtual Reality Surgical Simulation, and Objective Assessment of Surgical Competence and Training.

During his 25 years of military surgery he has been an active flight surgeon, an Army astronaut candidate, MASH surgeon for the Grenada Invasion, and a hospital commander during Desert Storm, all the while continuing clinical surgical practice. While striving to practice the complete discipline of surgery, he is aggressively pursuing the leading edge of advanced technologies to formulate the architecture for the next generation of Medicine."

Bio retrieved from the 5th Annual General Surgery Conference
http://gs.cme-ksu.org/publish/article_241.php

FOREWORD

Dr. Richard M. Satava, MD FACS

From the nascent beginnings of 'standardized patients' in the 1960's by Howard Barrows to this epic on virtual patients, the revolution in medical education continues to evolve. And while the concept of a standard, consistent actor for a specific disease in order to provide a reliable and quantitative training and assessment methodology is still the core component, the virtual patient might even be considered a second revolution within the 'standardized patient'. While it is true that a virtual patient will not provide as 'realistic' of an experience in the near future (though it may be possible a few decades from now – look at how 'realistic' many Hollywood 'special effects' movies are today), virtual actors will be able to provide a solution to a number of the limitations of today's standardized patient actors.

The science of simulation is the '800lb gorilla' of the Information Age, sitting silently behind the scenes as computers and the internet gain the attention. Yet it is simulation that can predict the future, reduce risk, improve efficiency, decrease costs, provide a variety that is not achievable in the real world and free the learner (and teacher/evaluator) from the constraints of time, place and cost. As striking as the accomplishments of real patient actors in training and assessment are, there are real limitations that impede a greater use in medical education. Real actors must be trained, they cannot truly exhibit the disease state (because they do not have the disease) and cannot provide the very wide variety of variations that disease states would present. Nor can they change sex, ethnicity or other cultural characteristics that provide a diverse exposure for the learner. Because they are real, they may not be available at a time that they are needed, (i.e. scheduling conflicts) and they are very expensive. They require space (a 'dressing room') to prepare themselves for their performance. And they require substantial time to be recruited, to be trained to exhibit a specific disease state, as well as trained to evaluate the performance of the learner.

Virtual patients, on the other hand, provide a number of advantages – which help solve some of the limitations above. And given the current difficulties with the 80hr workweek (potentially soon to be even less hours) that lessens the time available for the learners, the increasing cost of space, salaries, and time, having a virtual actor residing on a computer, available at any time (and from any place over the internet) without any substantive additional cost above the initial investment, provides a substantial cost and efficiency benefit. In addition, a library of virtual patients with multiple variations of the presentation of a disease type, in many different cultures and for both sexes, increases the richness of the experience of the learner.

Although the fidelity of the virtual patient will continue to increase, it will not replace the real patient actor in the near future; however implementing virtual patients can get the learner 'higher up the learning curve', so when the real actor is used, the learner will receive much more benefit from the encounter. In addition, because virtual patients are computer generated, it is possible (and will likely begin to be implemented in the future) to automate the assessment as well as the training scenarios. And if you are in agreement with the Dreyfus model of skills acquisition, once basic competence is achieved, it is through exposure to a large number of variations that moves the learner up the scale on skills acquisition to proficient, expert and master. Providing such variety in the real world of real actors in real simulation centers with real faculty is cost and time prohibitive – but certainly achievable in virtual environments.

This prelude is simply to illustrate the power that virtual patients can add (not totally replace) to the already proven value of standard patients to the scholarly training and assessment of medical students, nurses, residents and the full spectrum of healthcare professionals. The relevance of this book is that this is the first comprehensive and 'full cycle' monograph that addresses the above issues in depth through the use of virtual patients. Not only is the monograph academic, but it is also practical. And there is underlying all of the discussion and illustrations, a true sense of creativity and innovation – this is not a simple rehash of previous work (i.e. connecting the dots), but rather it is 'discovery of new dots' as Steve Jobs is fond of pointing out . The following are some of the examples of the broad scope that is covered – it is 'simulation writ large' – as applied to training and assessment of healthcare professionals.

The book begins appropriately by defining not only what standardized patients and virtual patients are, but also the supporting instructional infrastructure necessary to understand value (and limitations) of these surrogate patients – concepts such as problem based learning, machine learning, scenario thinking (planning), case-based reasoning , the Dreyfus model of skills acquisition, etc. It addresses the practical issues of how this infrastructure can be instantiated in a virtual patient. In addition there are accurate juxtapositions of virtual vs. prerecorded vs. real patients and when each are best used, as well as the importance of immersion and presence in the training experience. Other nuances are elucidated, such as choosing the appropriate level of fidelity of the 'actor' to match the level of training for the learner or of the challenge of crossing the 'uncanny valley' between obvious low resolution graphic representation of a virtual patient to the high fidelity replication of a real patient, as well as clearly explaining the current technologies in the softer aspects in the representation of virtual humans such as emotion, visual fidelity, gesture, posture, pose, gaze, body motion, nonverbal cues and interactivity , to name a few.

Virtual actors are getting 'smarter'. There is a review of the significant progress in artificial intelligence research, with breakthroughs occurring principally in cognitive neuroscience and synthetic thinking. The full power of fuzzy logic, continuous variability, deictic context, and conversational logic being combined with advances in human social, behavioral and cultural (HSBC) research has resulted in virtual humans with emotive behavior, personality traits and motive – they are beginning to appear to have perception and cognition. While scripted actors have served in the past, the advanced research herein points to a new generation of virtual actors that are demonstrating some elements of artificial intelligence, though they certainly cannot pass the Turing Test yet.

Along with reviewing the above advances in developing virtual humans, there is an excellent review of the importance and fundamental role of acting and drama to creating an actor/teacher which has credibility to the learner. In addition there is inclusion of the impact of social media, and how it is adding to the revolution in the way education is provided and the importance of 'social influence' in capturing attention and incentive to excel – experts, celebrities, friends, crowds, etc. There are even references to improvisation, twitter and the TED Conferences and how they are contributing to the change in educational paradigm.

The monograph ends with creative speculation on the future directions of standardized patients (virtual and real), with the incorporation of video gaming techniques and technologies, holograms, gesture technologies and next generation artificial intelligence

There are sufficient and appropriate illustrations, graphs, figures and images to enhance both the understanding and the enjoyment of reading about this intriguing new science. It is likely that this monograph will become a standard reference for the development of virtual patients and will also contribute to the growing understanding of real patient actors as well. I hope that other researchers will gain the amount of hard scientific knowledge as well as enjoy reading this monograph as much as I have.

1

STANDARDIZED PATIENTS

A Standardized Patient (SP) is a trained actor who portrays a particular illness to provide training to medical students and professionals. SPs primarily use written scripts and additional paper-based training for preparation of practical and board exams. Medical institutions use various methods for training such as hiring preceptors for reenactment of scenarios, viewing archived videos, and computer-based training. Currently, the training that is available can be enhanced to improve the level of quality of standardized patients. This book will be examining current processes in standardized patient training and investigating new methods for clinical skills education in SPs. In addition, other areas that will be explored will be case studies for Standardized Patient training, Rating and Reliability, Virtual humans in SP training, conversational agents and models, Inter-Acting, the fundamentals of acting, and future technologies that can be leveraged on for standardized patient training.

When it comes to training, the modality that is selected can possibly affect the performance of the actual SP case.

STATEMENT OF THE PROBLEM

Effective and accurate training is needed to enable Standardized patients (SPs) to be concurrent with the medical technology and training objectives that are constantly changing. The training that is currently available has not evolved much, and this evolution is needed for the future growth and sustainment of training. Existing training can now be supplemented with simulation, artificial intelligence, and virtual worlds. The use of Standardized Patients in role-play training to learn clinical skills and medical interviews has been existent since 1963 (Rossen, 2010). A typical standardized patient interaction includes a role-playing scenario that lasts five to thirty minutes (Rossen, 2010). When this interaction occurs, questions are asked from the physician or medical students based on the medical case that is learned from the SP (Rossen, 2010). The medical student or doctor interacts with the patient and gives them a diagnosis based on the physical and verbal cues that a patient provides (Rossen, 2010). Standardized patients are actors who are hired to portray a patient who possesses a particular medical condition (Rossen, 2010). These SPs perform this same type of role-playing task with several different students and must act consistently to maintain the integrity of the curriculum and standardized board exam (Rossen, 2010). Attaining this skill to be able to successfully resemble the same patient and scenario with each student is essential to providing a standardized training solution. This standardized trait is especially needed when evaluating students. This role-play interaction, aside from being used as a training component, is also used as an evaluation metric for the Step 2 CS (clinical skills exam). When interviewing a few medical students, the conclusion that was gathered is that the result of passing is not as significant as failing the Step 2 CS. If the board exam is failed, it can be very challenging to enter into a reputable or any residency program. Another issue is that some standardized patients lead the student on with answers. This could potentially provide an unfair advantage to some students. In short, a successful SP interaction and clinical skills assessment should have SPs that are standardized.

A major responsibility of a standardized patient is to be able to portray a patient with the fluent knowledge of the symptoms; and also be able to properly rate the medical student after the interaction. Rating is done by accurately completing a Standardized Patient checklist. Having the standardized patient effectively reenact the scenario in an identical standardized manner can be a challenge.

When comparing the actual verbal content to the accuracy, there is a difference. If you take the verbal content responses, they are correct within a 90.2% margin of correctness, while the accuracy comes within a 30% range of accuracy (Tamblyn, 2009). Some areas where some of the standardized patients can improve are: remembering how to respond correctly when a medical student asks questions, understanding what is asked, and being able to interact effectively and consistently (Rossen, 2010). There are moments where the questions or combinations of questions could be unexpected or unable to be comprehended (Rossen, 2010). The diversity of a medical student can create an area for error as well, as some individuals may have different accents in language, diction, and delivery. The VERG (Virtual Environments Research Group) at the Computer Information Science Engineering Department at the University of Florida has developed a Role-play trainer which trains SPs to utilize the voice logs of previous medical students to assist in clinical skills education (Rossen, 2010).

The tool that is created can provide the standardized patients with a broader array of questions that could be asked by a medical student, preceptor, or physician. The training lies in being able to provide the correct responses to the particular questions that were asked, providing an appropriate response, and giving a form of feedback to answer what is asked. A more optimized solution in simulating the conversation that is delivered by the Virtual Human allows the SP to have a better level of proficiency in a standardized patient interaction (Rossen, 2010; Wessell, 2003).

Fussell (2009) speaks of a community-based treatment organization using SPs to portray a substance abuse client. In order to reach a certain level of expertise, SPs in this scenario trained for 15 to 25 hours (Fussell, 2009). A good amount of this time consists of tasks regarding memorization and periodic assessments of the material that is presented (Fussell, 2009). What if there was a better way to do this? Furthermore, what if this better method engaged the user more, had tools to track performance, and got smarter as more users used it?

Another instance of SP training is when another educator was used to assist in training SPs on a psychological case. This case interfaces with a virtual human that represents a realistic representation of physical and psychological symptoms (Fussell, 2009). The areas that are required for the SP to perform are created and built into the learning tasks of the training system. This system is good at being able to pinpoint the areas that could potentially be an obstacle for reaching a particular level of proficiency (Fussell, 2009). A focus group is used to evaluate the validity in portrayal of these cases. Experts in the areas of these learning applications are asked to observe these experiences. The chosen subjects were tasked with giving a particular score on a checklist for each SP. The scoring was based on the Likert-Scale. The questions are based on different types of factors on the interactive experience such as how realistic it is (Fussell, 2009).

MULTIMEDIA AND PART TASK TRAINING

Multimedia is widely used as a method of training. Frequently, when learning modules are examined, the scope of the tool needs to be considered. The question that is often asked is whether this tool is used for assessment or training. After assessing the objectives and goals of the experiment, the learning module that is developed for this experiment can be considered a training tool. Part task training has been a popular form of training for critically focused skills. The reason for its popularity is because of this concept's success in reducing cost and training time. Heavy amounts of resources and unpredictable maintenance and costs are usually the outputs of a more expensive multi-functional trainer. This poses true especially when the task is very specialized. Part task training with virtual humans and immersive environments can assist in SP education. Certain developmental modules that are relevant to the desired educational needs can be selected. One example of a solution is an SP rehearsing a clinical skills encounter. These encounters can be set in a virtual and immersive environment. It is within this environment where a virtual standardized medical student can assist the SP in learning the lines of a clinical case. Further skill sets that could be developed with a tool are better proficiency of the case, and a reduction in anxiety. Occasionally, this anxiety is a result of the anticipation of a role-playing event. This allows the training to occur on-demand and in-situ; without having to hire complete faculty and additional resources. In other words, an SP can individually receive the focused training that they need to become smarter on a particular skill set. This training for readiness does not replace a standardized patient training curriculum, but provides a positive supplement which provides an overall cost savings over a long period of time.

While there are varying definitions of multimedia, it can be generally defined as "extending training beyond pure text using a combination of several potential media types such as graphics, animations, video, auditory, and photographs" (Conkey, 2010). "Indeed, technological advances continue to produce new media types that can be used in multimedia based training and educational venues" (Conkey, 2010). In Conkey's case, the experiment uses an integrated multimedia training tool for comparison of a machinima interface vs. pre-recorded skills when learning soft skills.

A question that is often asked in an avatar vs. video experiment is if avatars provide similar or exceeding results in training when compared to video delivery modalities. Avatars may not be aligned at the same level of fidelity and realism that the video provides. However, technology has greatly improved to provide a better quality of realism so that many of the gestures, inflection, tone, eye movement, and emotion can be represented with simulation software, algorithms, decision modules, and artificial intelligence. A definition of fidelity is "how accurate a system is able to recreate an output which is identical to its input" (Wordnet, 2010). Yorick Wilks discusses an initial prototype in his paper (2011) that has "information extraction techniques", "mixed initiative in dialogue control", and other interesting concepts for a companion that seniors can use. His project called COMPANIONS is in the EU and provides a method for a virtual companion to cultivate an adaptive association with their users. This type of bond that is shared allows the technology to learn the user's curiosities, feelings, and needs.

An electronic educational system should assist the user in achieving a mastery of skills that are needed to complete a task on the job. Training fidelity is essential in providing a robust educational solution. This solution should provide the user with an experience that is immersive and provides retention of a learning task. As seen in the screenshots below, the avatar to the right may not provide an exact replica of the character to the left, but what if the same training value is there?

Figure 1: Video/Avatar Screenshot Comparison

(Permission to use image granted by Curtis Conkey (2010))

In addition, since the avatar is used, synthetic voice matching technology could be used to modify the voice track and alter it to accommodate new learning tasks. This could provide extensive savings as it takes a great amount of time, cost, and collaboration to produce videos with human subjects. Cost savings could also be incurred when edits to the voice sound file could be changed. In addition, lip syncing can be used to match the alliteration of the character's speech. This lip synching technique allows the avatar to be reused to teach new content. This provides a better alternative to editing video footage of human actors for a brand new training scenario. However, a recurring question is if avatars react with the same amount of credibility as that of the video actors. Little, if any, research has so far compared avatar actors with human actors for their effectiveness in standardized patient training or performance assessments. There are many dimensions of human interaction and perceptions that can affect the production of effective avatar-based training (Conkey, 2010).

Conkey asks the following interesting questions: "Will the trainee have the ability to have an immersive experience (level of presence) while using avatar actors versus human actors?" "Furthermore, if the presence values are negatively affected, how will the training outcomes be affected?"

HOW ARE STANDARDIZED PATIENTS TRAINED?

There are various methods used currently to train standardized patients. Some training approaches utilize integrated methods, while others are more focused. The following sections below will provide details on different methods and comparisons on how SPs are educated. In addition, explorations will be made when comparing different modalities. From these discoveries, we will be able to see if there significant differences.

COACHING STANDARDIZED PATIENTS

One method of training standardized patients is coaching. A team is only as good as its coach, and the quality of the coach will indicate how well the performance will be (Wallace, 2007). In order for a case to be more valid, the SPs should be at a similar level of performance so that some people are not getting better training than others. It is essential to have good SPs, as this will show how well the interaction will play out (Wallace, 2007). It is not a simple task to make this role-playing production a success as a lot is involved when having a successful SP experience while still refining the coach's expertise as they go (Wallace, 2007).

While developing coaching abilities, there are some qualities that Peggy Wallace, the author of "Coaching of Standardized Patients", refers to as qualities of an effective coach. One of the first traits that are to be able to be knowledgeable is the realms of drama and leading actors (Wallace, 2007). Since the standardized patient experience is highly involved with patient portrayal, the coach must know something about drama to be able to properly train and simulate an actual standardized patient encounter. A second trait that is needed is to have trusting level of comfort with the SPs (Wallace, 2007). As quoted in Funke & Booth, "the relationship should be one of mutual respect, understanding, having love of the work, and also having trust" (1961). The coach must have a general foresight to how the case will be, and it is only after that visual image of the interaction that the true encounter will be able to come to fruition with the SPs (Wallace, 2007). A third trait is being able to provide an aspect of enthusiasm and benevolence to their work (Wallace, 2007). Bringing this imagination into the SP's mind is one of the key factors that represent patient portrayals. When a coach successfully demonstrates this skill, the SP is motivated to bring the patient case to life in its true essence. Finally, the fourth trait is to trust their intuition and what they know. This intuition must come from within, and they must use that to help guide them in their interactions. SPs and their coaches must also be intuitive in their role-playing and coaching so that they are able to think and act quickly on their feet (Wallace, 2007). Being able to duplicate these characteristics in training provides the ability to produce a quality curriculum.

To become an SP, the SP must be able to successfully show the traits of a sick person, evaluate the quality of a medical student, have a vision of the interaction in their mind, complete a thorough checklist, and provide suggestions and expertise to debrief to SPs and educators afterwards (Wallace, 2007). As mentioned before, the training on standardized patients is used to perform in any high-stakes clinical skills assessments. As a result, the SP must have a fluent knowledge of the case and be able to know exactly how to act and portray illnesses and characteristics successfully (Wallace, 2007).

Wallace also suggests that there are basic guiding concepts that are needed to be aware of when it comes to SPs. One of the things to be cognizant of are the knowledge, skills, and abilities that an SP must possess (Wallace,

2007). Another is to ensure that all the SPs understand what is meant by the word standardization. Standardization does not always mean that all the SPs need to act in the same manner, but standardization is better described as having the SP portray a patient consistently in his/her own rendition relevant to the scenario. Furthermore, standardization may mean something different to SPs who have acting experience. Actors who are training may have a perception that it may be a negative trait to make a scene standardized. There are some responses and gestures that are situational. For example, a medical student's inflection in speech could provide more expectations to provide gestures that supplement the words that are put out. Standardization can also be seen as an overarching interpretation. An interpretation of standardization that is commonly used is making training available to a large group of people. Having leadership among the SPs so that they all see the same view as the educators and coaches will help to attain this consistent vision and goal among the SP community (Wallace, 2007).

According to Win May, an essential aspect in clinical skills training is to have the SP be able to evaluate medical students at an above average standard. This means that when they rate the medical students, the SPs are giving an answer that is correctly graded. These rating grades must be attained at an accuracy of at least 85% or above (May, 2008). To ensure that this occurs, the efforts of the SPs can be observed by subject matter experts (May, 2008).

2

VIRTUAL HUMANS VS. PRE-RECORDED HUMANS IN SP TRAINING

This chapter will review a case study that compares a Virtual Human vs. a Pre-Recorded Human.

STUDY OVERVIEW

The scope of this research study was "performance assessment". This research method investigated if a Virtual Human could perform just as well as a Pre-Recorded Human for an SP performance assessment. However, a follow-on study can utilize SPs in pilot studies for the prototyping and testing of a commercialized SP training solution. Furthermore, SMEs could later be used to code the rating ability of SPs. This educational module tests the knowledge of an SP case, but is not intended to replace a standardized patient training curriculum. It is intended to serve as an additional clinical skills tool which reduces the need for extended use on more expensive resources or expenses in staffing to educate patient interviewing skills, medical knowledge, and remembering critical points of the clinical skills case. Furthermore, the focus is not to display a high fidelity human computer interface solution, or develop a simulated solution for training, but to leverage existing technology to show that virtual humans can provide learning transfer. This learning transfer should be similar to or better than traditional training with a medical expert, pre-recorded human, reading scripts, or structured didactic training.

TEST

The objective of the experiment is to investigate if a significant difference exists between the two groups: Virtual Humans and Pre-recorded Humans. The scores of both groups will be compared when participating in a performance assessment that tests their knowledge of an SP case. Subjects also complete surveys that analyze how useful the education tool was for its desired application, open ended feedback surveys, and the overall experience of the performance assessment. Research with 52 human subjects is necessary. Sufficient information could not be gained by other research not involving human subjects. The population consisted of working professionals and students of diverse skill sets and backgrounds. The main criterion was that participants were comfortable with being audio recorded and familiar with using basic computer functions. Another requirement that was established was that at least half of the sample population must be above 45 years of age. This sample population was justified by contacting several standardized patient educators from various medical institutions. When interviewing an SP educator at the Standardized Patient Program at a medical school in the Midwest, they said that they had SPs of all ranges from 18-80 years of age. However, the most commonly used were 50 and above. The Academic Program Manager for SP & Teaching Associate Programs at a Hospital in the Northwest was also interviewed. This group hired 2-month-old babies, 8- and 11-year-olds, young teenagers for teenager cases, and young couples who had a baby, but her average range was between the 45 and up range. Finally, an SP Educator at a local Medical College said that the average age is above 50, but they are now having more people in their 30s come in because of the economy and with people being more inclined to seek work.

As a result, the subjects were distributed in the mix as follows. Also below is the study design.

AVATAR
Ages 45 and up: 13
Ages 18-44: 13

TOTAL: 26 subjects

Pre-Recorded Human
Ages 45 and up: 13
Ages 18-44: 13
TOTAL: 26 subjects

Group TOTAL: 52

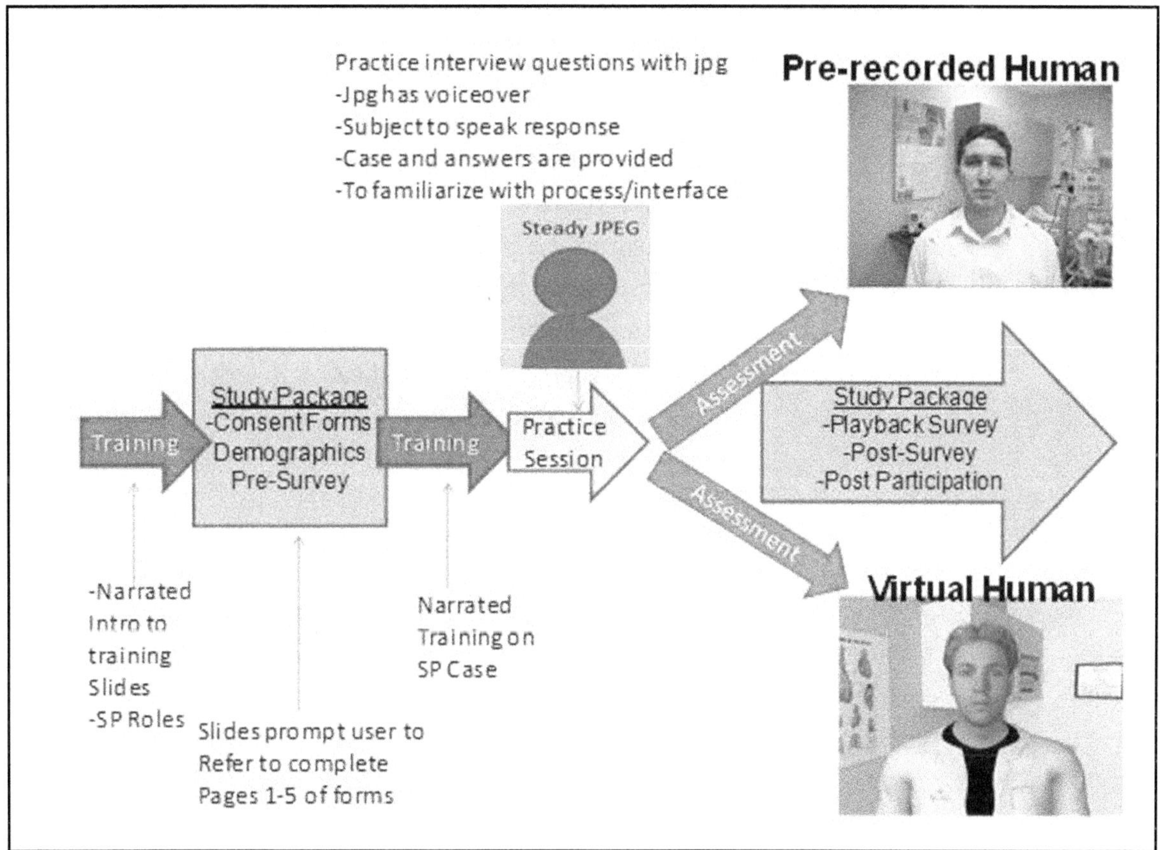

Figure 2: Study Design

(Permission to use image of Virtual Human has been granted by the METI Lab at the University of Central Florida www.METILab.com. Permission to use image of Pre-recorded Human has been granted by Scott Mercado)

The only manipulation in the experiment was in the performance assessment. In reference to Conkey (2010), a video training module was converted completely to avatars and the results showed that there was no change in results when comparing the two. The results were that it does not make a difference if you use video vs. avatars. Although that study used tasks in a hospital emergency room, the comparison seen in the two training modalities is valuable. Preparing medical students to communicate with patients who come from a variety of race, sexual orientation, financial status, age, and other considerations is very beneficial to medical students in assessing the patient in the most effective way.

SUMMARY OF MANIPULATION

This study manipulated whether participants performed differently when faced with altered modalities. This simulated a patient interview as participants were prompted to provide an answer upon each response of the conversationally modeled Virtual Human. The critical difference between the two conditions was the realism in the interaction. The avatars do not currently have the fidelity that compares to the realistic representation of a human image. This could affect the credibility that the participants are exuding, but the benefit is that this study provides the evidence that there are benefits, disadvantages, or no change based on the evaluation of the measurements provided.

POWER ANALYSIS

The one independent variable is a performance assessment modality which is at two levels: Virtual Human and Pre-recorded Human. Power must be collected after collecting data as it cannot be controlled with these types of tests. The chances of having better power can be created by having larger samples or having data that has a farther margin apart. However, to get a second opinion, a power analysis was conducted to make an approximation on how many participants are needed to provide enough power to analyze the data to sufficiently correspond with the hypothesis by utilizing software for statistical analysis G*Power 3 (Faul, Erdfelder, Lang, & Buchner, 2007). A statistical computer program like this allows the researcher to enter parameters of the study and then estimate the required sample size in order to detect a specified effect size. According to the use of G*Power 3 (Faul, Erdfelder, Lang, & Buchner, 2007), the medium effect size was at .04 with .80 power, which indicated a minimum n of 52. A similar study by Conkey (2009) estimated medium effect size in determining the number of participants that would be required. The participants are randomly divided into two groups for testing against the two major treatments to the training.

RECRUITMENT

As mentioned, the target number of subjects that are needed is approximately 52. The recruitment occurs by using the NAWCTSD bulletin board, flyers, bulletins and emails to university students. The complete study is done on a combination of a laptop, a PC microphone (as subjects are voice-recorded), and a paper packet that has paper-based measures. The Principal Investigator (PI) is standing by to provide additional assistance.

STUDY WORKFLOW AND TIMELINE

Upon the potential research subjects entering the study site, the PI provides each subject with an Informed Consent Document (ICD) and Privacy Act Statement. After informed consent has been administered and the ICDs have been signed by both the PI and the subjects, the PI provides a paper packet to each subject and introduces them to the computer-based training. The computer-based training directs them to the packets to complete. The packets include demographics and a pre-survey on their knowledge and confidence in standardized patients. After the forms are complete, the participants begin an instructional training session on standardized patient roles and a standardized patient medical case. This tutorial and case is based on the case that is present in the University of Florida's Virtual People Factory software. Within Virtual People Factory, a tool to train Standardized Patients was developed called the Roleplay Trainer. Brent Rossen, the developer of this tool, published a paper (2010) that discusses how the Roleplay trainer is used within VPF to be able to train SPs.

After the tutorial of SP roles and case is complete, a practice session occurred to allow the subject to be familiar with recording their voice, reviewing answers and the case to answer questions based on both, and navigating through the slides. The practice session asks 19 questions which add up to a total score of 38 (two points each). The same questions are then asked later during the Performance Assessment. The performance assessment is where the answers and case are not available to review while in the section and the subjects have to come up with the answer based on what they learned in the

Standardized Patient Training and practice session. After the practice session, half of the participants begin a performance assessment with a simulated virtual human (avatar). The other half perform with a pre-recorded human that is delivered via video. Both modalities have the same content, resembling a standardized patient interview. The character on the screen (either an avatar or a pre-recorded video) asks questions regarding the case. The subject is to verbally respond as if they were truly conducting an interview interaction. As mentioned, this time the subject is not given the answers or the case as a reference. Instructions are given in the beginning of the session as well. This interaction is recorded. After the recording, the subject completes a performance assessment experience survey on the usefulness of interactive performance assessment. After this is done, the subject then provides open ended feedback about the study such as strengths of the study, areas for improvement, and additional comments. Finally, a Post Survey with the same questions as the Pre-Survey and a Post Participation Form will be administered to the subject. The audio-recorded interactions of the subjects will be transcribed for single blinded grading. The scores of the population that used the avatar will be compared to that of the pre-recorded human.

THE TIMELINE FOR THE STUDY

1-Consent forms/Privacy Act Statement: 7 minutes
2-Pre-survey: 3 minutes
3-Training (learning about SP roles and the Case): 5 minutes
4-Practice Session: 5 minutes
5-Performance Assessment: 10 minutes
6- Perceived Ease of Use and Open Ended Feedback Survey: 10 minutes
7-Post Survey: 2 minutes
8-Post Participation Information: 2 minutes

TOTAL: ~44 minutes

REQUIRED EQUIPMENT AND SUPPLIES:

-Laptop
-PC microphone
-Audio recording software
-Microsoft Office with PowerPoint (prefer 2007 and up)

The scores of the correct responses of the practice session will be graded using a ranking scale of 0-1-2. 0 is used to represent the answer being incorrect, 1 for it being partially correct, and 2 for it being completely correct. The PI will be grading the assessments single blinded (all the data is transcribed onto a sheet, and is graded later blindly after all the data is collected without knowing which treatment each subject's data is categorized under). This is done by assigning each subject with an identification number. Funding was not available to hire other personnel to grade the papers.

These, along with the Perceived Usefulness, Open Ended Feedback Survey, and Pre and Post Surveys provide additional data that is represented from the study. To calculate results for these, we can use the T- test to see if there is a difference in the scores of the two groups.

OBJECTIVE/SUBJECTIVE MEASUREMENTS:

Dependent variables will be the scores achieved on the interactions based on a ranking of 0-1-2. A Two sample T-test assuming unequal variance is conducted. All subjects have a potential of achieving a score of 38 (19 questions x 2 points each). An additional analysis technique can also be used to determine whether an effect seen in the data is due to the manipulation of the independent variable or the result of random variation.

JUSTIFICATION FOR EXCLUSION OF SPECIFIC GROUPS:

An age restriction was that the research subjects must be at least 18 years old. Anyone with a history of seizures shall be excluded from participating in research involving the use of typical video and/or computer games. The PI will have responsibility for administering informed consent, briefing research subjects, scheduling research subjects, collecting data, conducting analyses, and writing report(s). Janet Raskin, a research assistant that was recruited for the assisting in the study also provided support in data collection.

DEMOGRAPHICS

The table below demonstrates the demographic pool of the subjects selected for the study. The age range was 19 to 68 with a mode of 22 (4 subjects out of 52 of age 22). A pilot study was conducted with 13 subjects to get familiarized with the data collection and overall study procedure. Subjects are very much evenly spread throughout the age. In Table 1, age distribution is categorized in three parts. The age group between 30 and 50 makes up for around 48% of the total subjects. The proportion between genders is not even but very comparable. The study is not inclined to any extreme side in gender. The Participants were predominantly Caucasian with almost 50% of the subjects. Following the Caucasians, were the Hispanics who represented about 21% of the population. The average assessment score seems to be spread evenly in all demographic categories. The only score that stands out is for the Asian race. The mean assessment for the Asian race is 30 with a standard deviation of 6. This indicates the high variation among the Asian group.

Additional demographic data was collected and analyzed in the following table to establish each participant's education level and knowledge about the study. All subjects recorded their education before the study and this data is used to further analyze the mix among subjects. The data for education level is collected into two parts where education of Masters and PhD level is considered as Advanced degree. About 36% of the subjects have an advanced degree and the mean assessment score is very comparable in this category.

Data is collected to capture proficiency levels in acting and healthcare experience. The subjects who responded with previous acting experience were around 27%. Similarly, subjects with healthcare experience were around 23%. The initial review of mean assessment scores between these categories indicates that their scores are very close and it seemed like their acting or healthcare experience did not skew scores.

DEMOGRAPHICS TABLES

Table 1: Modality, Gender, Race, and Age Demographics

	Variable	Frequency	Percentage	Average	Std Dev.
Condition					
	Pre-recorded Human	26	50.0%	33.5	3.0
	Virtual Human	26	50.0%	33.9	3.9
Gender					
	Male	30	57.7%	32.9	3.8
	Female	22	42.3%	34.7	2.7
Race					
	Asian	6	11.5%	30.0	6.0
	African American	8	15.4%	32.3	3.3
	Caucasian	26	50.0%	34.2	2.5
	Hispanic	11	21.2%	35.0	2.2
	Native American	1	1.9%	38.0	0.0
Age					
	Below 30	15	28.8%	34.9	2.3
	Bet^n 30 and 50	25	48.1%	33.2	4.1
	Above 50	12	23.1%	33.2	2.9

Table 2: Education, Acting, and Healthcare Demographics

	Variable	Frequency	Percentage	Average	Std Dev.
Advanced Degree					
	MS & above	19	36.5%	32.7	4.4
	BS & below	33	63.5%	34.2	2.7
Acting expe.					
	Yes	14	26.9%	34.6	2.2
	No	38	73.1%	33.3	3.8
Healthcare expe.					
	Yes	12	23.1%	33.7	2.6
	No	40	76.9%	33.7	3.7

OPEN ENDED FEEDBACK RESULTS

Participants of Virtual Human modality predominantly had the following feedback:

- Slow down the voice (70%)
- Less engaging/reality as you know it is not human (65%)
- Easy to understand (30%)

Participants to Pre-Recorded Human modality predominantly had the following feedback:

- Easy to understand and work (75%)
- Little rushed into the interactive process (45%)

HYPOTHESIS TESTING

The question being asked is whether there is any difference in the performance assessment score between training methods of Virtual human and Pre-recorded human.

The six step hypothesis testing is conducted as below (Corty, 2006):

TEST:

The question being asked is whether there is any difference in the performance assessment score between training methods of Virtual human and Pre-recorded human.

Variable		Frequency	Percentage	Average	Std Dev.
Advanced Degree					
	MS & above	19	36.5%	32.7	4.4
	BS & below	33	63.5%	34.2	2.7
Acting expe.					
	Yes	14	26.9%	34.6	2.2
	No	38	73.1%	33.3	3.8
Healthcare expe.					
	Yes	12	23.1%	33.7	2.6
	No	40	76.9%	33.7	3.7

Table 2: Education Acting and Healthcare Demographics

1) *Assumptions:*

- The samples of Virtual human and Pre-recorded human are independent as subjects are selected and assigned to training method randomly.

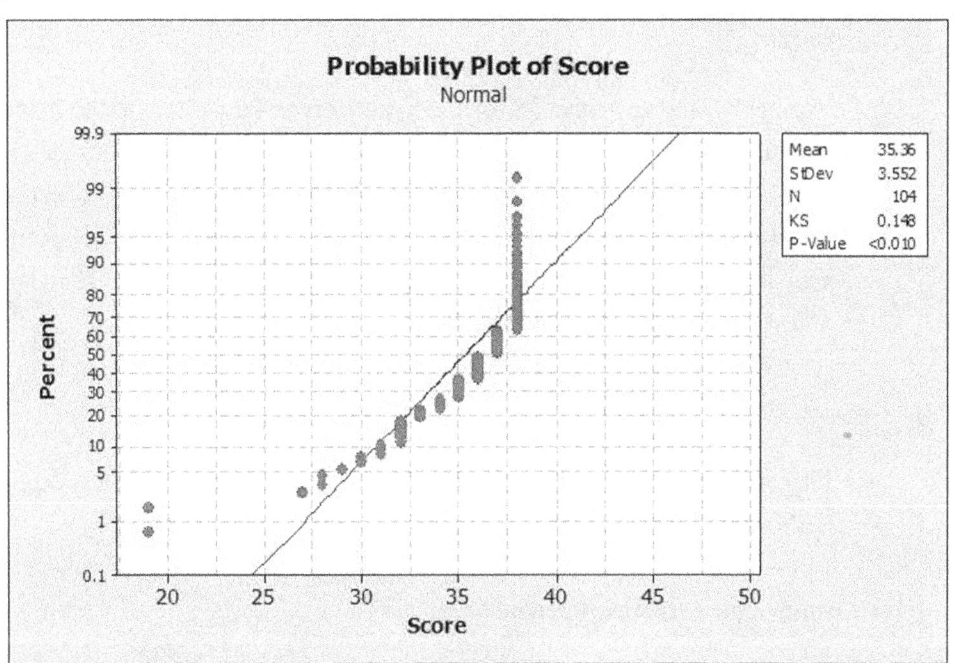

Table 3: Kolmogorov-Smirnov test of Normality

The partial descriptive statistics is listed below:

The standard deviation of both samples does not show big difference among them. The larger value of std dev. is not twice as large of the smallest std dev. Based on this, it can be concluded that homogeneity of variance is followed

Table 4: Training Method Homogeneity

Training Method	N	Mean	StDev	SE Mean
Virtual human	26	34.23	4.03	0.77
Prerecorded human	26	33.46	2.98	0.59

2) *Hypothesis*:

- There is a difference in two conditions (Virtual human and Pre-recorded human) when comparing the scores of a Performance Assessment in a

Standardized Patient case.

- H_0: Mean score of Virtual human = Mean score of Pre-recorded human
- H_1: Mean score of Virtual human ≠ Mean score of Pre-recorded human

3) *Decision Rule*:

- We are willing to make 5% of the Type I error so alpha = 0.05. If the p-value of the two sample t-test assuming unequal variances analysis is greater than 0.05, then that category is not significant. Furthermore, the mean difference is not significant, so we will fail to reject the null hypothesis. If the p-value is less than 0.05, then the mean difference is significant and we will reject the null hypothesis.

4) *Calculations*:

- Microsoft Excel 2010 is used for two sample t-test analysis, the output is shown below:

t-Test: Two-Sample Assuming Unequal Variances

	Virtual Human	*Pre-Recorded Human*
Mean	34.23	33.46
Variance	16.26	8.90
Observations	26	26
Hypothesized Mean Difference	0	
df	46	
t Stat	0.78	
P(T<=t) one-tail	0.22	
t Critical one-tail	1.68	
P(T<=t) two-tail	**0.44**	
t Critical two-tail	2.01	

Table 5: Results of a T-Test using Two Sample Assuming Unequal Variances

CONCLUSION:

The p-value for the two samples of performances assessment scores is 0.44 which is greater than 0.05 à **Fail to Reject Null hypothesis**. As a result, we conclude that the Performance assessment method of Virtual human or Pre-recorded human does not make a significant difference on Assessment scores.

After the analysis was complete, it was seen that there is no difference in standardized patient performance when comparing Virtual Humans to a Pre-Recorded Human. Although there is no change, this still shows value when using simulation. When the use of the Virtual Human simulation provides the similar results as the pre-recorded human, the Virtual Human is a better solution as it is more customizable, allows diversity, allows synthetic voice for different learning objectives, and is on demand. In addition, almost all aspects from the PANAS scale showed positive results; especially in Interest, Enthusiasm, and Proud.

DISCOVERIES

Some discoveries that were noticed were:

- Some subjects prefer using an Avatar because they feel more at ease
- Some subjects don't like the Avatar, because it is not as real
- Younger people like to use the Avatar because it is more similar to video games and is "cooler"
- One subject said that he didn't even focus on the avatar, because he was too worried about remembering his lines. He had a picture of the lines in his head instead.
- One subject said that when he looks at a character, he focuses on the background and if something in the background doesn't relate to the character he loses his focus
- -Some subjects reach for their back or stomach in real life when speaking to the avatar/pre-recorded human.
- Some said this was because it helped them remember
- Some said that it was because for a moment, they thought they were talking to it
- Some said it was to be in "character"

Below is a table that calculates the words per minute when comparing the two modalities. On the table, it can be noticed that the Pre-recorded Human has a higher words per minute count than the Virtual Human. The Virtual Human was purposely created to have a more synthetic sound compared to the Pre-recorded Human. The synthetic voice is good for testing the technology, but a more human-like voice is beneficial for high fidelity clinical skills training. Some examples of software that can be used are NextUp Talker, Cepstral, and AT&T Natural Voices.

Table 6: Virtual Human vs. Pre-Recorded words per minute comparison

Question #	Virtual Human Time in seconds	PreRecorded Human Time in seconds	Words	Virtual Human time in minutes	Pre-Recorded Human time in minut
1	1	1	6	0.02	0.02
2	2	1	6	0.03	0.02
3	2	2	7	0.03	0.03
4	3	2	9	0.05	0.03
5	2	1	5	0.03	0.02
6	3	3	10	0.05	0.05
7	5	4	18	0.08	0.07
8	3	3	7	0.05	0.05
9	3	3	7	0.05	0.05
10	4	3	10	0.07	0.05
11	3	2	11	0.05	0.03
12	2	2	6	0.03	0.03
13	3	3	7	0.05	0.05
14	3	2	9	0.05	0.03
15	1	1	3	0.02	0.02
16	2	2	5	0.03	0.03
17	3	2	8	0.05	0.03
18	2	2	6	0.03	0.03
19	2	2	8	0.03	0.03
Pauses between phrases	9.5	9.5	0	0.16	0.16
TOTAL	58.5	50.5	148	0.98	0.84

Virtual Human words per minute	Pre-Recorded Human words per min
148/.98	148/.84
151.7948718	175.8415842
152 wpm	176wpm

3

RATING AND RELABILITY

RATER TRAINING

Rater training is important when trying to understand how to rate medical students and assess their performance. Rating is crucial when understanding a standardized patient's responsibility to properly gauge a medical student's competence. A good form of practice is to have the SPs provide their response immediately after the interaction, while it is fresh in their minds (Wallace, 2007). This is an effective approach as there are several occasions where there may be a specific action that the SP performed that was not connected to every checklist response. An example of this is when an SP forgets if a student correctly pointed to where a particular pain is. If too much time has passed, the fresh memory and experience could fade, and the bias of the SP could potentially fill in the blanks (Wallace, 2007). This could conceivably cloud the true assessment of the role-playing interaction. The following pages discuss rapport, unreliability and bias in rating.

RATER RAPPORT

Understanding the user-centered and relationship-based approach to clinical skills and healthcare is not always clearly defined. As a result of the ambiguity in this area, there has not been much research that backs that the fundamentals of this concept are trustworthy (Hall, 2009).

An important factor that needs to be evaluated is the level of rapport that a person has (Hall, 2009). Second, it is important to forsee relations in the future that are relevant to rapport (Hall, 2009). Having this foresight is crucial to preparing for an interaction that can either be detail oriented or vague. A final important task is to come to conclusions after observing a quick instance of an interaction (Hall, 2009). Rapport is a quality that all members of a medical team should want to acquire and refine (Hall, 2009).

INTER-RATER RELIABILITY

Inter-rater Reliability is important when using different raters for evaluation of a standardized patient encounter. There are several different aspects that need to be analyzed. Inconsistencies can possibly be seen in areas where raters are required. Biases and standardization are issues that won't always be consistent, but results can be found out when studies are performed. The reliability studies in the following sections show examples of how inter-rater reliability is crucial in properly rating medical students for high stakes exams and clinical skills assessments.

BIAS AND POOR INTER-RATER RELIABILITY

An examination that focuses on neurological clinical skills is analyzed for bias and extent of inter-rater reliability. Residents were graded based on certain qualities and skill sets with the use of a Clinical Evaluation Exercise (Mini Cex). Some of the things in particular that were looked at were clinical skills, attitudes, and behaviors (Schuh, 2008). This experiment examines inter-rater reliability along with bias that is present in a Neurology Evaluation Exercise (NEX). The local faculty that does not have the sufficient training is observed to see if it behaves different than ABPN examiners that are not affiliated (Schuh, 2008). Furthermore, some other goals in this exercise was to see if the NEX scores were within a favorable comparison with the neurology residency in-service training examination (RITE) scores and to also see how many studies are needed for reliable testing and passing (Schuh, 2008).

Approximately four different departments were involved in the study and some demographical information was captured for research purposes (Schuh, 2008). Since it was important for the identities and experiences to be unknown, the residents were taught to be at a low competency (Schuh, 2008).

The sample consisted of thirty-two residents (21 men, 11 women) who were involved in the research (Schuh, 2008). 63% of the population, which is a larger majority, were PGY-2 residents (Schuh, 2008). The performance of the Pre-study for the RITE in 2006 was fluctuating throughout these groups (Schuh, 2008).

As the goal of the study was not to prove that the graders knew who they were grading, it was ok if some of the graders had some preferential treatment (Schuh, 2008). The more important scope of the study was that the faculty did not know how advanced or not advanced each of the residents was (Schuh, 2008). Even though the inter-rater reliability level was minimal, there was still a similar bandwidth of the range that fell within a 75 percentile performance. A videotaped session that was later debriefed to raters could be a valuable learning tool that would pose some training value. Modeling and simulation could also be used in this dissertation with applications of virtual humans and conversational modeling to replicate scenarios.

CAUSES FOR BIAS AND LACK IN RELIABILITY

Possessing requirements that are already pre-calibrated could affect the integrity of the rating (Tamblyn, 1991). This passage describes a study that discovers the origins of the unreliability. Two universities were involved in facilitating an identical SP test for clinical clerks in 1987 (Tamblyn, 1991). The study showed that there was a rating bias towards where the location of the test site was. Videos of the population sample were taken and it was seen that there was a reasonable range of reliability (.37 to .52) (Tamblyn, 1991).

However, the aspect of rater agreement did not have the same results (Tamblyn, 1991). Sometimes, an amount of partiality can be reduced by putting a particular framework in place to not allow the mind to give special preference to a particular treatment in a scenario. The following study delves into the comparisons of web-based versus traditional rater training.

ENRICHED RATER TRAINING USING INTERNET-BASED TECHNOLOGIES

An important component in training is producing high quality individuals who are able to perform consistently and effectively. This can be done with the proper instruction. Although this need has increased, a sufficient amount of research has not been performed to show enough data to support this. A potential reason is because a healthcare system has not completely adopted this yet (Kobak, 2006). When trying to gauge the performance of a rater, there are two traits that must be kept under close consideration. The first skill set that must be acquired is conceptual knowledge. The second is applied skills (Kobak, 2006). Conceptual knowledge plays a large part in understanding the way that scoring is performed, how things are done to scale, and how scaling is performed (Kobak, 2006). However, applied skills allow the ability to display how well an individual can conduct a clinical interview (Kobak, 2006). Even though both of these skill sets are expected, many individuals simply use training literature or a pre-brief with a subject matter expert in the healthcare arena. Kobak also mentions that 75% of the population applies paper-based literature or similar methods. However, this alternative is not advertised as the most optimized solution. Proper rater training is essential to the Standardized Patient community so that every medical student has a fair advantage of being involved in a standardized process of the clinical skills portions of their board exams.

To provide a solution to this gap in SP education, training, and performance, effective tools can be used to enhance the instructional systems design. This tool allows a user to stay consistently engaged (Kobak, 2006). A popular approach to assist in this is integrating the internet and didactic learning flow (Kobak, 2006).

Being able to preserve a traditional concept with a more engaging experience provides more returning users and an overall better tool (Kobak, 2006). A good indicator of success is to observe the user's activity and performance before the tool is used (Kobak, 2006). What is expected is that an enhanced training tool will provide better results. Many times, the enhancements can provide a significant alternative to the existing platform for learning (Kobak, 2006). Several applications now provide opportunities for the learning to be continuous through many channels (mobile phones, email alerts, facebook updates, etc).

4

VIRTUAL HUMANS IN EDUCATION

VIRTUAL HUMAN IMMERSION AND PRESENCE

Virtual Humans can be integrated into innovative and collaborative training solutions. These integrations can allow for an experience that brings them into a specific environment that is related to the training task at hand. They have the ability to bring the students into an environment where a new awareness of occurrences could happen (Privateer, 1999). During extensive periods of time, studies have applied concepts that are augmenting teaching with simulations that can result in increased learning and retention (Woodward, Carnine, & Gersten, 1988). One specific finding for students with low reasoning ability was that simulations offered a bridge to learning and understanding (Cox, Abbott, Webb, Blakeley, Beauchamp, & Rhodes, 2004). Simulations also show a great representation of how multiple entities can collaborate. This also allows educators and students to learn about models (Kolb, 1984; Kolb, Boyatzis, & Mainemelis, 2001; Montgomery, Brown, & Deery, 1997).

Immersion is when many of the senses are taken over with simulation, and the user feels as though they are part of the experience. The aspects of the simulation are a normal extension of their functions even though they are in a simulated or in a synthetic environment. Furthermore, when a user is able to interact with a mediated interface, it provides a sense of immersion.

Presence is also known as having the sensation of being at a particular location or experience (Heeter, 1992; Lessiter et al., 2001; Witmer & Singer, 1998). During this experience, a user is able to participate in an experience that has a realistic look and feel. In addition, they react when there is an activity that captures their attention (Heeter, 1992). Virtual Reality has been involved in simulating the stimuli of the human mind to bring in a certain level of presence.

FACIAL EXPRESSIONS IN COMMUNICATION AND EDUCATION

Humans are able to communicate with their face and language (Cassell, 2000). However, when combining facial expressions and gestures, new meanings can come into inception. Face to face conversation can be enhanced with facial expression and gestures (Nickerson, 1976). These communication aspects are things that can also be integrated into a human computer interface. An embodied conversational agent (ECA) is able to incorporate body movements, emotion, and model the functions of conversation that lay beneath the facial features. It is also important to understand the traits and reactions of a user to be able to properly model them. One thing that allows an avatar to relate to a homo-sapien is being able to decipher typical habits that they possess (Cassell, 2000). One example is when an ECA can serve as a tutor that can teach new lessons to a user, but still show relation and empathy towards the user's motives. This is especially impressive when the system develops a situational adjustment based on the user's emotional response or physical reaction.

A performative is a key indicator of intent of a speaker (Cassell, 2000). Furthermore, the performative suggests why the speaker is communicating when it comes to a specific topic (Cassell, 2000).

Facial displays can be used to indicate a certain feeling. When these facial displays are used in a particular way, they can replace certain words. Eye gaze is also an important tool in facial displays as they are able to control the level and location of a conversation. Computer Science groups have been able to create synthetic representations of these facial expressions and gestures in ways to assimilate to human behavior (Cassell, 2000). Gestures can be known to have unpredictable characteristics and are known as being the following: Iconic, Metaphoric, Diectic, and Beat (Cassell, 2000). Iconic gesture can resemble a particular perspective (Cassell, 2000). Metaphorical gestures can resemble a particular metaphorical symbol (Cassell, 2000). This type of symbol allows a better understanding of a concept such as a person rolling their hands together while saying the phrase "get the ball rolling" (Cassell, 2000). Diectic gestures take up a particular area and solicit cues. Beat gestures are small "baton like" motions can get the attention of a user and also provide opportunities to symbolize particular aspects of the conversation (Bavelas et al., 1929).

The timing of different movements in the eyebrows and forehead can also play a particular role in accenting the importance of certain words and messages. Some of these gestures have multiple functions (Cassell, 2000). For example, a smile could indicate happiness, but could also provide a good medium for social interaction.

STORY LISTENING SYSTEMS FOR EDUCATING CHILDREN

Justine Cassell's "Children and Technology- Story Listening Systems" book speaks of how the decisions to either allow children to use computers or not is a constant debate. Later mentioned in the book is learning based on play and also developing critical skill sets that computers can provide limitations to. However, with the new technologies of haptic and visual systems, these limitations can be minimized. Justine's system of a story listening system allows this type of play in an environment where the child is elicited to respond in a way that allows creativity and immersion (Cassell, 2012). Along with the story listening system, virtual peers can be used to also assist children in learning tasks and be involved in telling a story (Cassell, 2012). Furthermore, another development called an authorable virtual peer allows the students to configure the conversational agent to test outcomes of particular simulations of the avatar.

ASSISTING IN EDUCATING SIMPLE LIFE SKILLS

Virtual humans can also provide value in educating people how to perform simple tasks around the house. These tasks, often simple for the typical human, can pose difficulty for the impaired. The individuals who need rehabilitation or are elderly could benefit from a companion or virtual human that can remind them to take their medicine or perform a particular ritual that is required for their health and safety. When a consistent and reliable solution is available to do this, the customizability is what adds the most value.

5

CONVERSATIONAL AGENTS AND MODELING

DESIGNING EMBODIED CONVERSATIONAL AGENTS

One of the most important differences between an ECA and an avatar is that an ECA has a conversational model and is simply designed to possess the traits of a conversationalist. An ECA also has the ability to recognize particular cues (Churchill, 1999). A good natural conversation that an ECA has should be built on the behavior of a human-like interface; and a good indicator of its intelligence is its ability to engage a human (Churchill, 1999). An example of an interesting observation is if an ECA were to ask a question where the eyebrow would raise and the human would respond with a headnod as opposed to speaking a response (Churchill, 1999). Even though two conversations are never exactly identical, there are common habits in a conversation that can be used as a good path for conversation like: "interaction, responding to queues, waiting for a cue to speak, inflection, emphasis, and breaking away" (Churchill, 1999). A framework that is static but also dynamic allows the structure of the conversation to be flexible in its ability to interact with a user (Churchill, 1999). The system should also ensure that the ECA gives an opportunity to take turns in its interactions and also focus on the conversational functions as opposed to the mere sentence (Churchill, 1999).

An ECA was developed to give a user a tour of a house (Azerbeyajani, 1996). Inputs from different devices were procured with the use of input sensors (Azerbeyajani, 1996). The software that was used was called STIVE vision, which implements the use of recording devices to capture the realistic aspects of the images (Azerbeyajani, 1996). Data that is received is given a time stamp for documentation purposes and then processed into a module that analyzes the understanding of the information (Churchill, 1999). It later collaborates with an understanding module to determine the state of the conversation (Churchill, 1999). Another model was developed name REA. This model knows to generate a response after a speech act and gesture is made (Churchill, 1999). The generator that is used to understand the objectives of communication from a request formulator is called a SPUD generator. It uses basic knowledge that is programmed to determine the premises for interaction (Churchill, 1999).

Along with an input system, it is also essential to have an effective output system so that a good flow of conversation is framed in an organized model (Churchill, 1999).

EMBODIED CONVERSATIONAL AGENT ALLIES

Different aspects of conversational modeling should come together at the end to accomplish a common goal and vision. Scenarios and storyboards can be used to properly plan how ECA interactions can effectively occur (Cassell, 2000). The process can evolve as the general design could be vague, but then more low level details can be elaborated on (Cassell, 2000). These storyboards and general designs can later be converted into an initial prototype of the conversational model (Cassell, 2000). Some things that are also laid out of the agent in the design are the ECA's personality and nature of interaction in a conversation (Churchill, 1999). The scenarios also expect tasks from the ECA; and the ECA should also be pleasant to look at (Churchill, 1999). The ECAs can sometimes resemble a human, but do not necessarily always have to (Churchill, 1999). Sometimes the lack of human-like features provides an increased sense of ease with the subjects. Abstract shapes can also effectively take the shape of an ECA (Churchill, 1999).

TEAM BASED TRAINING

Team based training is critical when it comes to training objectives. Using a distributed system in a virtual environment like in Second life can create this type of scenario. Along with being an instructor in a virtual world, an instructor can also call on a colleague that can also assist in co-instruction for a particular class.

A virtual scenario was created to show how an ECA can assist in teaching to learn a particular task (Johnson, et al., 1998). There are a few things that are essential for creating an immersive world. One of the initial things that are needed is an effective simulation. Simulation is important as it controls the behavior and feedback of what is seen, such as VIVIDS which is discussed by Munro et al. (1997). In addition, a visual interface that runs over the engine must be pleasant to view (Rickel,1999). The requirements that are established up front to determine how realistic the simulation is become one of the determining factors when investigating how effective a virtual world is. Speech can be recognized and accomplished. However, when a system can comprehend the signals of speech, it is a very effective tool (Rickel, 1999).

Cognition in conversational modeling consists of three layers. One of the lowest layers would model general human intelligence (Newell, 1990). Tasks would be defined more in the second layer, and the third layer would categorize the knowledge within the domain. A domain can be updated to accommodate different learning tasks, needs, and lessons (Rickel, 1999).

The task-oriented module is where the collaboration occurs for different tasks and objectives (Rickel, 1999). In order for some of the events to occur in a natural fashion, the ECA may not always have complete control of the actions (Rickel, 1999). Semi-automated systems could assist in managing the overlap where an autonomous entity is needed.

Behavior is controlled by rules: Operator proposal rules are used to assist in setting the configuration for the users (Rickel, 1999). When implementing agents that are lifelike, good pedagogy is displayed (Lester et al., 1997b). Pedagogy is a way of best practice for an instructional approach. However, there are two issues when considering quality in instructional value. The first is deictic believability, which is having an agent realize the physical properties of the environment that it exists in. The second is emotive believability, which refers to an agent being expressive and also motivational to the user

(Lester et al., 1997b). Deictic frameworks are used to address these two aspects of believability (Lester et al., 1997b). A prototype was created to test the effectiveness of a deictic framework called Cosmo (Lester et al., 1997b). This agent teaches network routing mechanisms with the use of Deictic gesture, locomotion, and speech (Lester et al., 1997b).

The educational benefits to emotive behaviors are as follows: the agent showing empathy in the educational pursuit and a sense of companionship, cognizance of the student's performance and enthusiasm for the participation (Lester et al., 1997b). The student's problem solving activities drive the engine for this (Lester et al., 1997b). Some of these behaviors can be constrained within particular domains, can be triggered based on particular actions, and can be customizable as the pursuit continues.

COMMUNICATIVE TASKS

Communicative tasks can also be bound by the level of formality that is expected in an interaction (Poggi, 1991). These factors can also be driven by the expected goals and emotions from the conversations (Poggi, 1991).

EMBODIED CONVERSATIONAL AGENTS AND SIMULATED PERSONALITIES

Computers eventually serve as companions and assistants, and the extension from an interactive system caused by a mouse, keyboard, or handset could eventually lead to obsolescence (Ball, 1997). "An assistant" would be able to effectively comprehend different ways to deliver the same message and also be able to provide feedback (Ball, 1997). There are several instances that a human expects the same type of feedback from an ECA that it would from a human (Ball, 1997). Understanding the social impacts in conversational modeling assists in guiding the expectations that humans should have when interfacing with ECAs. However, conversational modeling in the ECAs can also improve to make this adjustment easier in transition. Emotion can be modeled in the ECAs so that they may accommodate different stimuli from the users (Ball, 1997). However, emotional and expressive behavior is still being developed to be successfully simulated in a high fidelity arena (Ball, 1997).

Emotional responses are established in two dimensions (Lang, 1995). Valence defines the positive and negative aspects of feeling, while arousal displays the intensity that is involved in a response.

A Bayesian network can be used to model emotion and personality (Ball, 1997).

This type of network is able to predict the potential for different outcomes (Ball, 1997). It is also able to display an organic representation of computer behaviors that are within a particular emotional state (Ball, 1997).

A psychologically aware system is able to analyze characteristics of the user and is also able to make judgments (Ball, 1997). A model of this is able to do the following: "observation (study the sensory input), assessment (using an algorithm to determine performance), using a policy component to determine relations, and behavior of the simulation (Ball, 1997)." The policy module makes judgments of the user's psychological state by analyzing the conversation (Ball, 1997). Emotionally diverse phrases must also be accommodated using this concept (Ball, 1997). Vocal expression carries a stronger influence than the text-based expressions that are delivered (Ball, 1997). Inside the network is an expression node which provides a relation to arousal, valence, and friendliness (Ball, 1997). Faster body movements can also cause more emotional arousal (Ball, 1997).

ECAS THAT PRESENT AND SELL

Presentation software has provided the need for more integration with ECAs that are intelligent (Andre, 1995). When integrating these assets into presentation software, the look, feel, and interaction can provide for a more attractive solution to instruction and content delivery. Having a synthetic presenter can provide an added dimension to the sales experience. The advantage to this presentation technology is that there is an on demand speaker who is always available to facilitate a crowd of individuals on learning a new concept, idea, or school of thought. An example of this was created. An embodied conversational presenter was called a Personalized Plan-based Presenter (Andre, 1995). The agent did have its own personality that was autonomous in the areas of gestures, idle time, and immediate reactions (Andre, 1995). In order to test this, a study was performed. Half of the subjects participated in watching a presentation that was facilitated by an interactive agent. The remaining subjects watched the same module with only audio along with arrows that highlighted important areas of interest, which lacked the gestures and expression that the ECA had (Andre, 1995). However, after analyzing the data that was collected, reading comprehension was not affected; but the expression and feedback of the users had a difference (Andre, 1995). However, confidence was not sufficiently instilled with solely the use of an agent. Teams of agents can also be used to teach a particular learning task or lesson. When initiating a design for a presentation, some things to keep in mind are dialog types, character roles, dialog contributions, and scripted behaviors (Andre, 1995). Agents can also enter the marketplace serving the role of a sales person. Microsoft Agent can be used for this (Andre, 1995). Along with a salesperson, other roles can be taken on such as a financier (Andre, 1995). When developing this type of solution, there are two types of personality factors that must be created (Andres, 1995). The first is Extroversion and the second is Agreeableness.

Many of these dialogs can be complex at times. To mitigate this, the goals must be broken down into simpler pieces. It is the central planning component that is in charge of this. The ECAs are autonomous for the most part, but there are events that can trigger the personality traits of it being either an introvert or an extrovert (Andre, 1995).

SMART AVATARS

The best way for smart avatars to be modeled to be similar to a human is to be connected to the synchronization of motion capturing technology, so that posture changes, reaching, pointing, grasping, etc., is applied (Badler, 1999). For gestures that are not similar to real life movement, alternate designs must be created.

When interfacing with an avatar, natural language processing can be used. Some words that are exchanged can be conditional based on the feedback. One example of this is if an ECA is cognizant that another ECA shows traits of being unpleasant or hostile, and knows to draw a weapon (Badler, 1999).

An example of this behavior can be seen in a virtual environment called Jack's Moose Lodge where there are five virtual humans who interface with each other (Badler, 1999). Some of the agents are able to be autonomous, while others have been programmed with certain behaviors (Badler,1999). This virtual environment serves as a platform for multiple users to collaborate on a certain task, communicate, and also sense one another's intentions with a response (Badler, 1999).

VIRTUAL HUMANS THAT ARE EMBODIED WITH CONVERSATIONAL MODELING

ECAs that are embodied with conversational models come to life to take on the role of the desired tasks that the designer creates. Many of them start with a simple wireframe, which outlines the basic shape of the character that is being portrayed. When these wireframes are embodied, there can be up to thirty-three parameters of movements in the jaw, lips, and teeth that can be manipulated (Massaro, 1977).

Speech is another topic that is integrated into the design, and when considering speech, the inflection in the voice, pitch, and patterns play a significant role in how messages can be perceived.

The advancements in natural language processing have developed slowly, but the challenges still exist in fidelity, speech understanding, speech recognition, and lag in processing time of messages.

EVALUATING INTERACTIVE SYSTEMS WITH EMBODIED CONVERSATIONAL AGENTS

Interactive systems and new technologies that leverage the technologies of the ECAs are important, but developers still must determine why and how they are used (Sanders, 1998). Metrics should be put in place to track the progress and growth of these technologies (Sanders, 1998). One method is to compare a technique across other platforms and see if some of the needs overlap. Two things where this can apply to with Standardized Patient Training is the correctness of an SP evaluation form and the time to complete a training session. Testing and Evaluation has been also proven to be an effective method to document progress and growth (Sanders, 1998). Periodic reviews can also be held to document changes and action items. The end user drives the requirements for design, and the applications of systems engineering can assist in requirements development. Sometimes requirements can be ambiguous or out of scope, and these applications provide issues when considering the requirements for how and what would be desired to be tested. These user driven requirements can also affect the software that is created when the requirements change due to a change of high level objectives or realignment within the organization (Sanders, 1998).

ETHNICITIES IN CONVERSATIONALLY MODELED VIRTUAL HUMANS

One of the benefits to standardized patient training with embodied conversational agents is being able to implement diversity. Diversity can be seen in ages, sexes, races, and geographic locations. Sexual orientation, religion, and many other distinguishing factors can cause an individual to be considered a minority in a particular social group. ECAs don't have an actual race, nor do computers. However, when ECAs can represent a particular ethnicity, a user can interact differently based on the ethnicity of the agent and the user. Furthermore, when someone is part of the in-crowd, they are considered more socially attractive (Lee, 1993; Stephan and Beane, 1978).

USING MIXED REALITY WITH VIRTUAL HUMANS

Mixed reality is the integration of simulated components with that of the real world. The way that users engage with this can show how effective a virtual human encounter can be when it comes to learning particular skill sets. Johnsen explains a study in his paper that compares the effectiveness of an interaction with a user that interacts with an avatar on a life-size depiction as opposed to an avatar on a computer screen. The interaction study showed that users who dealt with a life-sized virtual human were more engaged than that of the user that interfaced with the virtual human on the computer screen.

HUMAN CENTERED DISTRIBUTED CONVERSATIONAL MODELING

"Human Centered Distributed Conversational Modeling" reduces the complex efforts of designing a conversational model with the assistance of an application called crowd sourcing (Rossen, 2009). The new knowledge that is created from crowd sourcing is generated from the operating person's inputs. This new information provides opportunities to educate with the VH conversational model. One of the first steps in HCDCM is to collect a mass of stimuli to begin with. With this sample, a domain expert guesses what is said to the VH; and then later approximates the response of the VH. Later, novices provide responses in the same fashion which gives new stimuli for the VHs. Later this is peer reviewed by a subject matter expert and validates the use of it.

A browser-based interview GUI allows an easy interface for communicating with the virtual human using a text to speech functionality. When matching items in the corpus, Virtual People Factory (VPF) uses a special approach that can recognize similar responses and elicit feedback accordingly (Rossen, 2009).

The Editor GUI is a domain where experts can create new questions and use VPF to interact with the use of phrases (Rossen, 2009). A web-based version of VPF allows the user to communicate with a patient with the use of an instant message-based interaction. (Rossen, 2009). Simulated clinical interactions that rely more on voice activation than text to speech are applied with the use of an *Interpersonal Simulator* (Dickerson, 2005).

BOOTSTRAPPING THE CREATION OF VIRTUAL HUMANS FROM EXISTING ONES FOR SP TRAINING

Virtual Humans (VHs) can be applied to the training curriculums of several applications. Some popular areas where they can be useful are in military training, patient interpersonal skills, and medical interpersonal training applications. Many training modules have had an interaction where the user interacts with a virtual patient and this practice session provides a great deal of part task training to master communication skills and bedside manner. Rossen's paper is quite interesting as it mentions the developmental efforts and time it would take to create new roles for each VH, and how this can be mitigated by using existing conversational logs from previous preceptors to assist in training SPs. This can provide a great training on teaching standardized patients how to rate. After an interaction is observed, they can complete a standardized patient checklist, and those results can be compared to that of a subject matter expert rater. This technique of using the utterances of a human from an interaction to create a new VH that can take on the role of the human is called bootstrapping (Rossen, 2010). A Role-play trainer that was mentioned previously in the Virtual Human vs. Pre-Recorded human study was created to assist in training standardized patients. The Role-play trainer is still the web-based interface, but can be brought to life with integration of the interpersonal simulator. However, there is significant back-end coding that needs to be done to accommodate this.

One of the difficulties that the Role-play trainer faces is that when it creates a question asking VMS from the logs of the VP - Medical Student interactions, there are issues being able to have it say the proper questions in a logical order that flows similar to natural language. This developmental tool serves as a layer that works above the existing Virtual People Factory website architecture (Brent, 2009). The Roleplay Trainer Creator is used to create models of conversation that works properly with the Virtual People Factory (Rossen, 2010).

A pilot study was performed to test how well the trainer worked on some users (Rossen, 2010). Surveys were used to get feedback on how well the pilot worked with users (Rossen, 2010).

PARTICIPANT MOTIVES IN COVERSATIONAL MODELING

It was often believed that the developer was expected to create a system that made the user content, which is still true. However, now the user can also assist the developer with feedback for new creations in software development. Halan mentions that internal interactions can be applied to help in this user motivation. This same school of thought can be used as a proof of concept in SP training. SPs may have a hesitation in the credibility of a training system as it is a rather new technology that may have not built the desired reputation that matches up against a live role-play training scenario with a medical student. However, their feedback can still be crucial in designing a system that is tailored to their learning curve and addresses the obstacles that are presented in learning a task. Leaderboards, narratives, and deadlines have been used as great tools to gather attention and motivation; especially in social networks and media. However, the issue is that many of the medical professionals have very limited time (Halan, 2010).

Narratives were used to capture attention of the user and describe the patient's background information and were used as part of the user interest emails. When a Deadline is pushed against the user, there is greater sense of urgency and motivation for the user to comply with the policy on time or earlier for attending the medical alert (Halan, 2010).

VIRTUAL PATIENT INTERACTIONS

Foster's paper discusses possible integrations of Virtual Humans in psychiatry educational applications. Aside from Standardized Patient training, standardization can also be a challenge in other areas such as psychiatry. A Virtual patient provides assistance when there is a need to simulate an interaction. Below are some images of the interactions that were used for training.

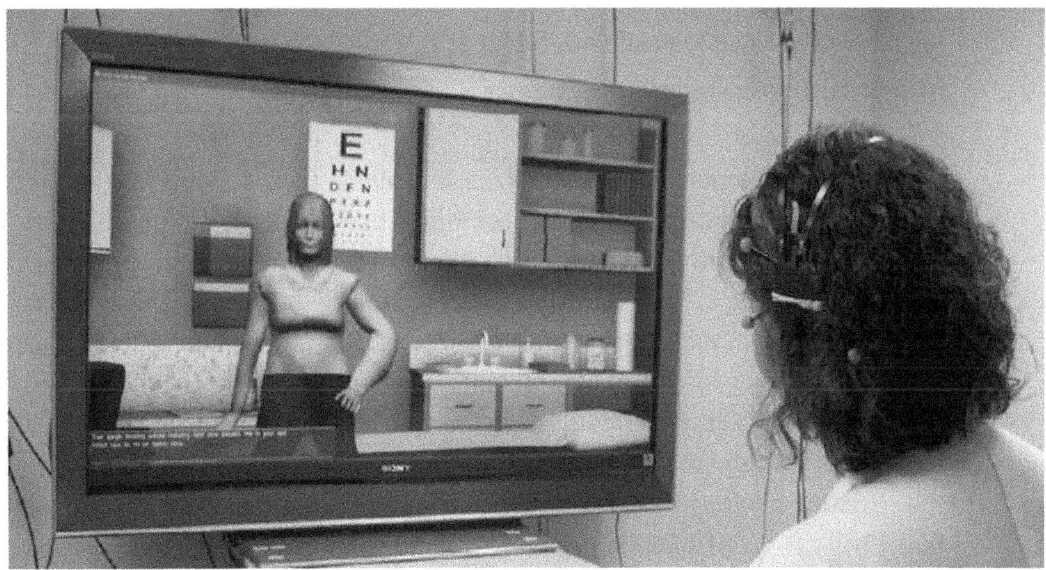

Figure 3: Life-size Bipolar Virtual Patient

(Permission to use image granted by Georgia Health Sciences University, (Foster, 2010))

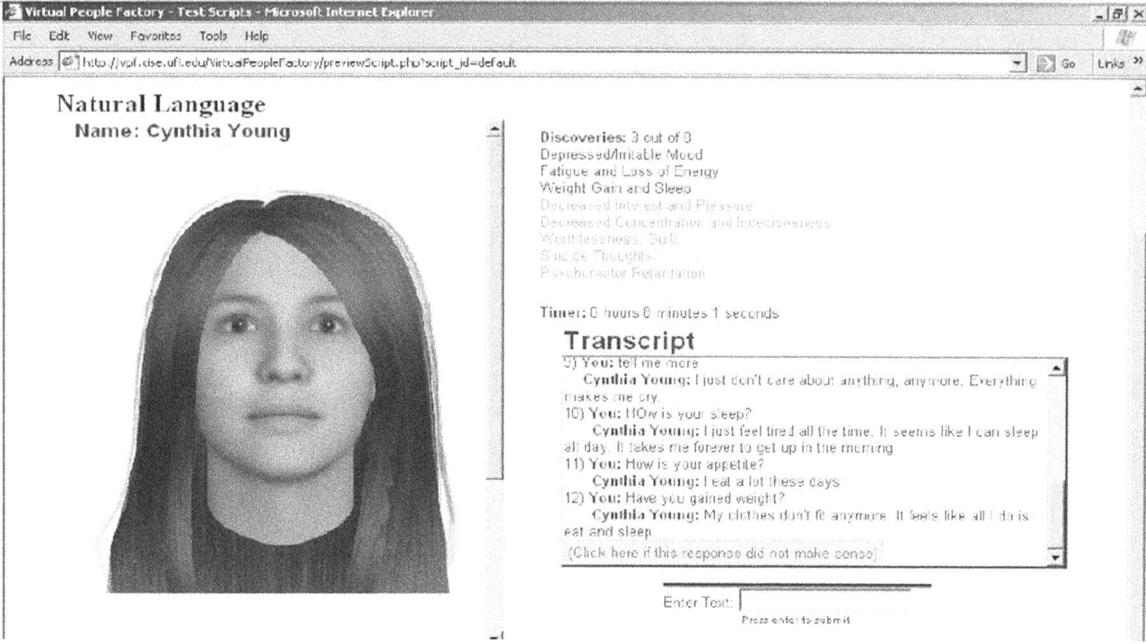

Figure 4: Web based Virtual Patient

(Permission to use image granted by Georgia Health Sciences University, (Foster, 2010))

One of the deficiencies in Standardized Patients is their memory of the case along with remembering the proper responses that are needed to provide a viable and realistic interaction. Some types of immersive training can be used to assist in memory. An application that can possibly be leveraged is a Virtual Reality Memory Training as explained in the article by Optale (2009). This simulation assists in addressing memory loss in the elderly (Optale, 2009). Virtual Reality is an experiential interface where there is a sense of being at the place where the experience has been established (Optale, 2009).

When modeling Virtual Humans, being able to break down the process into Five Levels of Hierarchy allows the decomposition of a problem into subsystems so each portion can be approached one at a time and can later be integrated into a consolidated solution.

VIRTUAL HUMANS PROVIDING MENTORSHIP

Mentorship is a widely important goal among many organizations. The valuable lessons that leaders have acquired and passed on to new protégés allows the protégés to become mentors as well. Embodied conversational agents can also become mentors (Sims, 2007). According to Lester (1997), motivation in people to learn can be enhanced. Virtual humans can provide support and motivation through the use of modeling and simulation. Role-playing actors can be beneficial in standardized patient training as they can pose as a standardized medical student that interacts with a Standardized Patient who is in the process of learning a medical case. However, in order to perform as a successful mentor, they need to effectively model the behavior of a successful mentor (Sims, 2007). Essentially, this type of smart avatar would be able to make decisions, inspire, and lead development as a real mentor would.

MENTAL MODELS AND IMMERSION OF THE FUTURE

If the time is truly taken out to understand what is distinct about humans, we can see that humans have the distinguishing characteristics to make themselves unique in several ways. These differences range from general ones such as gender and ethnicity to interesting ones such as being able to champion technical advancement and have distinct ways of wearing clothes. However, the true distinction that can be noticed by humans is the ability to create mental models. Ancient civilizations have implemented mental models that are similar to that of the modern day technologies that we have today for information technology, communication, and entertainment (Kurzweil, 2003). A very primitive form of virtual reality is the telephone. The telephone allows one person to communicate with another as if they were in the same room, when actually speaking from a distance (Kurzweil, 2003). Advancement in this area has now expanded to provide immersion in virtual worlds, and Kurzweil mentions that these virtual worlds are integrated into our contact lenses and woven into our clothing, so that the concept of computers as stand-alone systems are obsolete. Nanobots can also be used to intercept interneural signals to allow a human to enter a virtual world. Nanobots can also be used to perform surgical procedures to complete tasks while entering through natural orifices. It is also suggested by Kurzweil that by the year 2030, websites will be fully immersive experiences where emotions and experiences can be archived, and humans can increase their thinking with nanobot technology, which are constantly enhanced with biological and nonbiological thinking. Kurzweil also notes that in the year 2030, we will not be able to tell the difference between biological people who have projected themselves into a fully immersive environment. One of the most crucial factors for success in virtual humans is not only the level of complexity in technical advancement, but the realism and fidelity of the expressive characteristics. It's these characteristics that evolve into a personality.

TRUSTING VIRTUAL HUMANS AND SYNTHETIC THINKING

Ethics and standards are policies that should be regulated as a safety precaution when it comes to relying more on conversationally modeled humans (Plantec, 2003). This can pose a risk as virtual humans are given more social responsibility and influence to the extent that it could possibly take over the boundaries of a live human (Plantec, 2003). The issues of the future that Plantec suggests are the increased dependence of virtual humans in the future as humans not only rely on them for completing tasks, but as companions, lovers, and confidants. There are also assumptions that humans will one day rely more on the company of a virtual human for comfort than a real human. When understanding consciousness and the quantum theory, Hameroff and Penrose suggests that the brain can process 10 ^17 operations a second. Machines can process language at the unconscious level as much as we do. However, real organic brains use fuzzy logic which can accept inaccuracies and ambiguity; while computer brains are based on properly calculated algorithms based on rules which provide the illusion of a conscious personality (Plantec, 2003). However, a simulated organic brain that uses logic based on a fuzzy approach might provide a solution that would have some initial traits of a real brain.

ARTIFICIAL COMPANIONS

Yorick Wilks' book "Close Engagements with Artificial Companions" has specialized in various research efforts that involve the concept of companionship in artificial mediums. It evaluates whether they exist in virtual humans or simply a conversational model. It explores if artificial entities will later take on legal responsibilities, and are more existent in software applications than in robotic form. One thing that must be taken into consideration when developing these artificial interfaces is thinking beyond the capsule that carries the technology. This capsule embodies much more than a function to simulate something, but it is a true psychology that must be modeled. A question that is asked is if a growing population of this trend of virtual companionship will ever be as much of a challenge of that of a real population problem (Wilks, 2010). The better the technology gets, the more challenging it will be to succeed in a Turing Test. A Turing test is a test that compares how smart an intelligent system is when compared to that of a human. The originator of this test was Alan Turing, who in 1950 wrote the paper "Computing Machinery and Intelligence", in which he asks the question if machines can actually think. This question is hard to define because thinking can go back to the philosophical statement by Descartes: "I think, therefore I am".

FALLING IN LOVE WITH VIRTUAL COMPANIONS

Wilks' powerful book mentions the ethics and issues with humanizing robots. When robots and artificial humans are created as equals or entities that have legitimate responsibility in society, there is the possibility of dehumanizing people. This will happen if a robot is not seen as a tool created and owned by humans. These types of thoughts and approaches could be results of fears of the machine revolution of the future.

Along with the fear, there is also the fantasy world of having a relationship with a robot. Wilks refers to a book written by David Levy titled "Love and Sex with Robots". In this book, he mentions the concern that people could sometimes prefer an artificial relationship with a robot as opposed to one with a real human being.

WHAT DO VIRTUAL HUMANS THINK OF YOU?

Going back to the question, "do robots really think?", we think of the logic that is implemented to design an embodied conversational agent and understand that the decision modules and thought processes can almost simulate an instinct. In Justine Cassell's book "Embodied Conversational Agents", she explains how to model emotion and personality. When taking this to a deeper level, it can be evaluated if the virtual human can truly empathize and be sensitive to a human's thoughts, feelings, and responses. When looking at this, there truly is a perception that a virtual human has of us. Although this is designed through complicated computing, this designed perception is still a perception. The interesting thing to see is if this smart system will have the ability to be flexible with different personalities as humans are able to.

6

LEVERAGING SOCIAL MEDIA TO ENHANCE SP TRAINING

REVERSE MENTORING IN STANDARDIZED PATIENT EDUCATION

In SP training, mentoring of standardized patients is quite important. It is an essential supplement to role-play training and lessons. Traditional mentorships require a person who is getting started to have an individual that they can look up to. When a person has a successful mentorship relationship, they are able to look up to influential leaders but they can also serve as mentors to more junior personnel where they can share the new lessons that they learned to be positive examples for future successors.

However, a new approach to mentoring can be adopted. This approach requires the mentoring from younger professionals to more senior professionals. As it is now the information age, many younger generations are adopting social media as a regular platform for entrepreneurship, business development, and current events. The older generations who are more seasoned in their experience may not have as much exposure to these technologies due to commitments, responsibilities at work, and ties to family. As a result, there lies a gap in the situational awareness of emerging technology. Along with that, the social perspective of the new trends, schools of thought, and strategies are all valuable to learning new skill sets.

SOCIAL PROOF

Another novel area that reverse mentoring can help the senior and SP community with is the concept of social proof (Social, 2011). A proof of concept that can help validate that there is an impact to a particular concept is through influence. When an influence can be created, a following can be developed. A very inspirational TED (Technology Entertainment Design) lecture given by Simon Sinek explains how people influence. He presented a very interesting model that shows how successful entities like Apple, the Wright Brothers, or Martin Luther King have influenced large masses. His model has three words (why, how, and what) that describe the common pattern of influence. It is the "why" that shows a leader purpose in believing in to do something significant (Sinek, 2011). For example, when people who are hired believe in the same things that a leader does, then a successful influence can be achieved (Sinek, 2011). Simon was also able to translate how this communication from the inside out relates to biology of the brain (Sinek, 2011).

Now with different start-ups growing and a development in new technologies, it is quite important to be able to capture attention from an audience. This type of phenomenon is known as social influence. This can be used in gaining attention to training in a particular group. One example is a line that is formed in front of an event. Many venues use this method of capturing attention from the crowd. People who are passing by will see the line as a group of people who belong to a particular social group and could potentially be exclusive. This exclusiveness is a method of drawing a desire for a person to be part of something unique. Another example was listed in Social (2011), where a restaurant was able to increase sales by a percentage of 13-20% by simply highlighting particular items as the most selected choices.

Social (2011) lists Social Proof into five categories. The first category is social proof that is done by an expert. This method captures an audience by providing insight from an expert in a particular field. Some social media sites are now able to capture which users are the most influential by monitoring how many followers these users have, how much popularity, likes, or comments their statements receive. As a result, these people are individuals who can set a trend in a particular market. This is very powerful, especially when it comes to awareness of a particular topic of interest. Some other ways to influence are by using celebrities, user feedback, crowds, and feedback from friends (Social, 2011).

BLOGGING

The word blog stands for the words web and log (Blog, 2011). Blogs are great for building a community of followings based on a particular topic. Bloggers could be heavily used in the Standardized Patient community so that lessons learned on educating SPs could be shared. Difficulties that are faced could also be shared so that it does not happen on a constant basis with other educators. In addition, particular techniques that were successful in learning transfer for SPs can also be provided in the community of medical educators.

When not sharing a particular subject with a group, blogs can also be used for two other main purposes. One is for daily postings where a person can share their insights on a particular area of expertise. The areas can range anywhere from telecommunications technology to medical technology. Another application can be for advertising (Blog, 2011). A particular blogger can be hired to market the brand, the user friendliness, and benefits of using the product. An added feature could be to make the blogs more interactive (Blog, 2011). Underneath the blogs, users of a particular subscribed periodical could leave comments and discoveries that are relevant to the post (Blog, 2011). A similar example can be like on www.facebook.com, where people are able to leave comments under a wall post (Blog, 2011). Blogs can also be represented as videos (vlogs), art blogs, and mp3 blogs (Blog, 2011). Microblogging also involves multiple posts that are provided in a continuous fashion (Blog, 2011).

TRENDING ON TWITTER

A trending word is a word that has been posted many times on the social media site twitter. This topic is usually posted several times due to a popular topic, event or controversy that is currently occurring. Understanding these trends and being able to incorporate them into modern learning methods and technology will bring educators up to speed and awareness on fresh educational approaches. Social media is gaining momentum in terms of requirements to assist in marketing new technologies. Many firms are now looking to track which individuals can influence a group of people most successfully on social media sites. To accommodate social influence creators, these firms will often provide airline accommodations, hotel reservations, and admission tickets to events where particular vendors of interest are present so that when these individual's use these products, the digital crowd will follow. That is at least the hope that social influence provides to these advertising firms and vendors. This can simply be done by using internal metrics and tools to track who has the most followers, posts, and which profiles show indications of influence. Many of our world's leaders have been successful as a result of their ability to influence. This power in influence can empower a group of people to do phenomenal things, but at the same time can be used for harm. However, the aspect of empowerment that is in the scope of this book is to enhance clinical skills education.

TED (TECHNOLOGY ENTERTAINMENT DESIGN) CONFERENCES

As referenced before, these conferences are very inspirational and have various topics that are covered. These conferences have different categories, some of which are related to medicine, where comments can also be placed underneath the video. Being a part of this community and opening discussions with other subject matter experts will also increase breadth in a certain area of technology. If attendance to the local events is not possible, there are several local TED events that are made available to local cities called TEDx events. Each local region has requirements to view a certain number of lectures a year, and provide commentary to stay active. If a local chapter is not in a particular area, TED can be contacted to establish one.

SUBSCRIBING TO REAL SIMPLE SYNDICATION (RSS) FEEDS

RSS feed are also a helpful tool to be able to gather information on a topic of interest. A user can choose any particular topic and there are short descriptions of a particular subject. An RSS reader can be downloaded to a PC and to a mobile phone to have access to these feeds. When subscribed to these feeds, the user will receive several short summaries that briefly describe the topic which is updated very frequently. When the short summary is chosen, the summary will often expand into a full article. A good set of RSS feed subscriptions for an SP educator could be "Standardized Patient Training", "Modeling and Simulation for Training", "Clinincal Skills", "Standardized Patient Educators", "Learning Transfer", and "General Teaching Methods". These RSS feeds can be subscribed to on a smartphone, or on the internet via PC. Smartphones now also have the capability to directly share the feeds to twitter, facebook, and email.

BUILDING A COMMUNITY AND NETWORK FOR STANDARDIZED PATIENTS

Building a community of experts in the field of Standardized Patient Training expands your network that much more. It creates an organization that can also provide you with support. To fulfill the requirement for a medical focus group for my PhD, I reached out to the Association of Standardized Patient Educators. The organization was very helpful, and they assisted in collaborating with a team of SP educators to help me answer questions regarding utilizing simulation in SP training. Also on the organization's website (http://www.aspeducators.org), there is a "resources" section that provides some useful information on further educational opportunities in the realm of clinical skills and SP education. Listed below are some SP Training books recommended by the website (Association, 2011):

"Training Standardized Patients to Have Physical Findings" by Howard S. Barrows (1999) Southern Illinois U.

"Stimulated Recall (Personalized Assessment of Clinical Reasoning)" by Howard S. Barrows (2000) Southern Illinois U.

"Assessment in Health Professions Education" by Stephen Downing and Rachel Yudkowsky (2009) Routledge.

"Recruitment, Retention, and Training of African American and Latino Standardized Patients: A Collaborative Study" by Mauritha R. Everett, Win May, Carolyn Tressler Nowels, Deborah S. Main.

"Training Standardized Patients to Give Feedback to Medical Trainees: The State of the Art" by Patti Hatchett, Carolyn Haun, Linda Goldenhar.

"Quality of Standardized Patient Research Reports in the Medical Education Literature: Review and Recommendations" by Lisa Howley, Karen Szauter, Linda Perkowski, Maurice Clifton, Nancy McNaughton. Medical Education (2008) 42(4):350-358.

"Coaching Standardized Patients for Use in the Assessment of Clinical Competence" by Peggy Wallace (2006) Springer.

"Following the Threads of an Innovation: The History of Standardized Patients in Medical Education" by Peggy Wallace.

Attending conferences are also an essential venue for successful networking. These forums are great areas for new topics of interest to be shared with the community. Integrating this information on social media will provide the best vehicle to transfer this data. A great way to share this information about a new area of interest in research is to submit papers during a call for abstracts or proceedings for the conference. If the abstract gets accepted, then the author will get invited to speak about it through a presentation or participate in a panel discussion.

7

THE FUNDAMENTALS OF ACTING AND DRAMA

THE GENESIS OF ACTING

It can be said that it is almost instinctual for humans to act (Dolman, 1949). Although several people have not pursued a professional role in acting, there are several instances where people use the imagination to take themselves to a place of fantasy or even allow themselves to dream of being in someone else's shoes (Dolman, 1949). It may be as extreme as comparing humans to monkeys, where what is seen is done as a mimicry, but there are some motives in acting that do trace back to historical origins (Dolman, 1949).

One of the initial ways to learn is by natural imitation (Dolman, 1949). From a biological perspective, there are several living things that learn from imitating (Dolman, 1949). Primates, birds, and even young children learn from seeing others do (Dolman, 1949). The didactive motive shows a need for teaching through acting where primitive groups used it to initiate people into religions, traditions, and social customs of particular tribes (Dolman, 1949). This motive is the most relevant when it comes to SP training.

Many elder members of tribes would dress in clothing to represent tribal heroes or gods to represent the importance of the initiation (Dolman, 1949). A totemic ritual called Terrorization uses masks to imitate scary figures to scare young men for initiation (Dolman, 1949). Terrorization was also used in warfare to scare their enemies (Dolman, 1949). Finally one of the most popular motives for acting is Entertainment. This dates back to Shakesperean and Medieval times where dramatizations were held in theaters and jesters were called upon to provide comedic relief.

TRAINING AND COMMITTMENT FOR ACTING

One thing that is crucial to a standardized patient is having a firm grasp of acting concepts. Ed Hooks has recommendations for concepts in face acting. They are as follows: "The face expresses thoughts beneath, acting is reacting, know your character's objective, your character moves continuously from action to action, empathy is audience glue, and interaction requires negotiation."

One of the largest areas for improvement that is needed in SPs is the ability to act credibly. As a result, the next few chapters will provide some basic concepts of acting to help SPs gain a better knowledge and refreshment of techniques that can help an actor get more in touch with their character. As mentioned previously, most SPs are retired professionals who have little or no acting experience. The remaining population of SPs range from a broad age group that is driven by the need in the particular training task.

There is also an issue with an actor being a professional actor. When very committed actors play a role, they often stay in character to truly embrace the character that they must become in the next few months or even years depending on how epic the production may be. There was a very interesting article of the very talented musician, actor, and comedian Jamie Foxx. The article was titled "Man of Many Faces". This article discusses the commitment that Actor Jamie Foxx has had in his particular acting roles. When he auditioned for "Ray", he had to lose serious weight, as his frame was that of an athlete, by reducing his calorie intake (Smith, 2011). However, being conscious of his diet and consulting with nutritionists helped to make this possible (Smith, 2011). For some other roles he had to gain weight (Smith, 2011). But the largest factor was his commitment to the role. That type of commitment can also be applied to SPs, even if it is not as intense as changing the physical appearance for a role.

However, in some other cases, there are some residual effects. In SP training for highly emotional roles, residual effects can similarly be present. In a study performed by McNaughton, 16 SPs participated in a pilot study where they would be involved in an SP scenario which was an emotionally complex and intense role. In the pilot study, 11 out of the 16 subjects claimed to have remaining psychological effects that were based on information from a questionnaire that was completed by each of the SPs (McNaughton, 1999). After this pilot study was complete, four focus groups with 9 SPs each were video recorded and transcribed. After these scenarios were transcribed, 2 raters reviewed these samples (McNaughton, 1999). The conclusions were that some of these SPs indicated that there were remaining psychological affects that occurred even days later. However, there were some variables that distinguished the differences of these cases (McNaughton, 1999). So understanding these causes for these emotional effects can provide a better selection of SPs, acting techniques, and a refined ability to role-play and improvise in not only an intense role, but a simple role as well (McNaughton, 1999).

The feedback that was given from educators who have worked with professionally trained actors was that the role might be dramatically overdone. There needs to be a happy medium; where the SP truly represents the sickness but is still constrained to the boundaries of the medical scenario. To address this gap in SP education, the next chapters will focus on techniques for acting along with some fundamental concepts in acting and role-playing.

DUAL FUNCTIONS OF AN ACTOR

An SP has several responsibilities. They are not only required to portray a patient, but are also required to evaluate a patient by filling out a checklist. In doing this they also serve as an educational tool. However, as an actor, they also have dual responsibilities (Doleman, 1949). An actor serves as an artist and as an instrument (Doleman, 1949). As an actor serving as an artist, the canvas is the voice, body, gesture, facial expression, and emotions (Doleman, 1949). However, the actor as a whole is an instrument for performance (Doleman, 1949). As an instrument, the actor is known as a representation of the character and should essentially be able to be replaced by another person to complete the same task of portraying a particular role (Doleman, 1949). However, an artist is different as an actor in an embodiment and representation of the character that is desired to being played (Doleman, 1949). It is not of guidance for the actor to go against the director or any creative direction of the play, but simply for the actor to enhance and bring the character to life (Doleman, 1949).

ANALYZING THE PART

In acting, there is a part of a role that must be worked up to. According to Albright, one of the first steps is to consider the entire acting experience as a whole. What should also be analyzed is what does the scenario mean to the actor, and what is it composed of? When understanding how a play is designed, they can better place a perspective on how they fit in with the big picture. It is also important to visualize in advance how your character will look, act, and react to particular situations. Some other things to visualize are how you will look in particular physical positions, postures, and stances. Some things to use as a reference can be the actual play, descriptions in the beginning of the play, and footnotes.

Emotion

There isn't an actual scientific definition for emotion, but in the acting world it is based on the instinct. The raw emotions come from within, and when in its primitive form, it can be released through physical and extreme means. However, over time as human beings have become more refined, they have learned to control emotions and even express them through a pen and paper. An important question was that if the actor should actually feel their part. A response was given by Coquelin that the actor must still remain the master of himself throughout the most impassioned and violent action on the part of the character which he represents; in a word, remain unmoved himself, the more surely to move others (Coquelin, 1881, Doleman, 1949). An actor that lets the role take consumption of their being shows affect in the performance of the show along with causing stress on the audience and the cast. One example of this is the curse of "the Joker" character in Batman Movies. Rumors were spread that the role of the Joker caused quite an amount of stress to Heath Ledger which lead to his demise. Although there were speculations, there are several instances where the emotion in a particular character can consume the actor.

MOVEMENT

After analyzing a part, this mental image can be used to generate a mental model of how a physical movement is generated as an output of the visualized role. Pantomime is the act of communicating particular ideas to an audience with only movement (Albright, 1959). One major rule to movement is that there should be a productive reason for each of the movements to better supplement the dramatization (Albright, 1959). It should contribute to the performance, and the movement must be committed with no hesitation (Albright, 1959). Any type of movement plays an influential part in the interaction. When it comes to a medical representation, each and every movement has a significant symbolism to a sign and symptom. To be able to successfully provide a credible representation of these gestures, a healthy body must be maintained. The proper types of conditioning, flexibility, and presence are also needed to prepare for actively participated roles.

SPEECH

An essential characteristic of speech that Albright makes is that the speech must sound like a normal person speaking the phrase for the first time. It should not sound forced or rehearsed. This natural flow is important to provide a credibility of a character. As mentioned earlier in this book, one of the largest criticisms that medical professionals had with SPs was that the SPs didn't actually sound like they were convincing enough to be a sick patient. In order to speak naturally, the actor must also truly understand the lines and what they mean. Another crucial part to speech is being able to take the understanding of what the words in the line mean, and grouping them properly (Albright, 1959). Word groupings are very important and strategic, and the way that they are grouped can change the meaning of the phrase (Albright, 1959). Certain annunciations can accent particular parts of the speech and can also provide for an expected delivery. Not only are the word groupings important, but making things sound natural in a package of words is just as important (Albright, 1959).

Furthermore, aside from simply reading, the words should also reflect how the actor feels at the moment (Albright, 1959). The thing that an actor needs to be careful about is using a particular tone that does not match the expectations of the character. The lines that are said should truly be expressed with conviction. This conviction should display a clear image of what is expected. Also, when replying back to other characters the response is held with confidence and natural transition.

VOICE PRODUCTION

Having a clear sounding voice is essential for the SPs to be able to portay the patient. There are some fundamentals of voice production that can help preserve the right vocal tone. The vocal tone is created through the larynx, which pushes air from the lungs through tight fins called the vocal chords (Albright, 1959). When breathing, the chords are at ease, but when speaking they condense to make vibrations (Albright, 1959). These vibrations are resonated and translated through a recognizable vocal tone (Albright, 1959). This vocal tone is finally shaped to form words through tools called articulators (lips, tongue, jaw, etc…) (Albright, 1959). Similar to a string instrument, the tightening and loosening of the chords provide different changes in pitch (Albright, 1959). As a result, it is important to take special care of these chords by refraining from putting too much strain on them. The best techniques for voice production are from exerting air to the vocal chords from the diaphragm and not the chest. When accompanying this deep breathing with the regulation of abdominal muscles, a controlled voice can be achieved (Albright, 1959).

The articulators that were mentioned before are used to clear categories of sounds such as vowels, consonants, and whether the voice is coming from the nose or from the mouth (Albright, 1959). Many singers are taught to sing from the diaphragm. The issue with singing that takes away from the performance is if the voice becomes either nasal or from the throat. These two types of breathing take away from the diaphragm and requires training to master.

Consonants assist in giving mechanics, texture, and clarity while the vowels provide vividness and strengthen the words (Albright, 1959). Some exercises for relaxing, breathing, vocalization, articulation, and pronunciation are encouraged in assisting to build a better quality in speech for SPs (Albright, 1959).

EMBODIMENT OF A CHARACTER

Sometimes it is just as important to know the details of a character as it is to know the general motivations and attitude of one. These attributes contribute to the entire embodiment of a character and how it reacts to others in the play. It is important to not characterize them as part of a general group, but as an individual. An example is if the character is a fireman. The fireman would act like what people know of how a fireman would act. This in turn would be considered a way to develop the character to integrate into the set. Furthermore, it is important to not include natural traits of yourself into the character if it is not the nature of the character. This can take away from the character and possibly stray from the objectives of the character. To truly feel the character, it must go beyond the scope of the theater, and the actor must recall personal experiences that provide motivation to the feeling and expression of the character. These experiences can also be derived from social groups and families (Albright, 1959). An example of using this as a tool is to think of a very sad point in your life to help motivate and develop a character that is part of a very sad scene. However, the questions that are commonly asked are how close do they need to carry these connections? The answer that Albright provides is that it should be "deep enough to arouse an audience, but not too deeply lest he lose his 'self-control'".

Stanislavski believes that a trained actor should be able to portray a character and display the expressions at every performance. These expressions should also be able to be recalled at will. An often routine example of this is being able to cry at will. This can be helped by utilizing the imagination to visualize how the character actually feels and truly feeling the being of the character. When this visualization in the mind occurs, this artificial reality is believable by the audience.

MEMORIZATION OF LINES

Different actors vary in learning styles (Albright, 1949). Some are fast learners, while others require constant repetition. It is important for the SP to be realistic to those skill sets and tailor their learning approach accordingly (Albright, 1949). Furthermore, after this recognition of learning style is established, the studying of the role should begin as early as possible (Albright, 1949). An ample amount of time should be incorporated to be able to learn the character and be effective in working up the part (Albright, 1949). The commitment to the theater should also be realized and the lines should not only be learned during the rehearsals. As a result, these lines should be memorized and practiced before and after rehearsals (Albright, 1949). This practice and level of comfort are what will allow the SP to effortlessly role-play a particular character with credible expression and no hesitation.

It is wise to develop a study plan. However, this plan should be strategic to the time that is spent and should also be highly concentrated on without distractions (Albright, 1949). The time that is spent should be as constructive as possible. The study time should be allocated in segments of time rather than a large time period. A recommended amount is approximately two hours at a time (Albright, 1949). When a long practice session is performed, it can often lead to exhaustion and lack of energy (Albright, 1949). This energy is needed to continue training throughout the weeks to come, so a proper conditioning plan is preferred.

DRAMA-BASED EDUCATION

Drama-based education, which is one of the critical parts of SP training, is so valuable because it adds the human element to education. It also adds the critical role of improvisation. Improvisational drama will be spoken about in greater detail as it allows participants to respond (Wagner, 2002). Furthermore, the use of drama improves such characteristics like thinking, oral language, reading and writing (Wagner, 2002). Twenty-five studies show that drama correlates to improved oral language. Furthermore, five literature reviews verify that drama also assists in better reading comprehension (Wagner, 2002). The Whirlwind program is an organization that promotes reading comprehension through drama, and there was a study that was conducted that showed that fourth graders showed progress in reading comprehension three months earlier than other students (Wagner, 2002). Furthermore, drama has also provided a benefit to writing. Seven statistical studies showed that the quality and maturity of writing was greatly increased with the coordination of drama (Wagner, 2002).

PLAY IN CLINICAL PRACTICE

By definition, play can provide a means for four elements. They are known as: "nonliterality, positive affect, intrinsic motivation, and flexibility" (Krasnor and Pepler, 1980). Consequently, pretend enactment uses fantasy and surrealism to create an environment that provides a sense of ease. Play is used in clinical practice for many applications. A common application is utilizing it for coping mechanisms. There are simulation technologies available now that employ digital immersive encounters to allow soldiers to reenact a traumatic experience so that they may condition themselves to recovery. Many soldiers come back left with several factors that can cause residual stress. Technologies can now be leveraged to allow new types of solutions to prevent this. Another solution that allows play is a technology that amputees use. This technology allows the user to be in a serene, simulated environment that keeps the mind off of the recovery and allows the stress level of the patient to be at ease. Play is often used in therapy for children who suffer from post-traumatic stress and childhood conduct problems, when a traditional approach for recovery cannot be used (Russ, 2011).

ZONE OF PROXIMAL DEVELOPMENT

SPs can learn in a particular zone of development by what Vygotsky called the "lure to learn". Particular zones of development can be referred to as the domain where people are acting a particular scenario. For an SP, it would be within the constraints of a simulated patient examining room. For a construction scene, the constraints will be at a work site. Being able to successfully improvise within this particular zone of learning and engaging with the other members of the interaction will allow a fluid dynamic in interaction. The difference between drama and a story that is heard is that drama integrates words with body and gesture. With children, this technique can be adopted before learning to read and write. Primates are also able to use gestures and sign language to communicate with humans. As infants, all parts of making sense of the world is rationalized through the use of gestures, whether it be to eat, be changed, be comfortable or held (Wagner, 2002). Vygotsky refers to these types of gestures as the earliest types of communication. Gestures can become empowering when particular gestures are iconic.

CONSTRUCTIVIST THEORY

Constructivist theory suggests that human beings develop a customized learning process for how the world operates (Bruner, 1990; Wagner, 2002). This is developed not only through the physical representations, but also by reflecting and observing how communication is developed throughout the world. Constructivist Jerome Bruner provides three representations that gestures can relate to how human beings think. The first is enactive representation (Bruner, 1990). This thought process indicates that we learn by doing (Bruner, 1990). In SP training, a large part of the education is to participate in several role-play interactions with preceptors and medical students (Bruner, 1990). Iconic representation is done by knowing particular educational objectives through images (Bruner, 1990). These images are usually mental images that are developed to assist in learning transfer and build fluency in a particular drama-based learning exercise (Bruner, 1990). Finally, symbolic representation understands the actual meaning of a learning objective (Bruner, 1990). These representations are usually used to represent something that it originally isn't by using a symbol to provide recognition of it (Bruner, 1990).

VIDEO RECORDING AND PLAYBACK FOR SP EDUCATION

The level of technology varies based on the school. However, it is beneficial for SPs to see how well they performed during a certain interaction. Video recording equipment can assist in providing playback of progress and educators can highlight and track areas where improvement is needed. Some schools have very complex computerized technology that is connected to servers, and others have very basic recording systems which can be proven to still be as effective. The innovative and cutting edge technologies are the ones that use interactive technology to engage users for a simulated scenario. These scenarios can be recorded and can be practiced several times as the characters in the role-playing scenario are standardized.

USING DRAMA ACTIVITIES TO MEET COURSE OBJECTIVES

The educational potential of drama is used heavily in training for English as a second language. According to Dodson, the following six objectives are focused on using various drama activities.

1. To integrate reading, writing, listening and speaking
2. To improve pronunciation
3. To learn about the history and conventions of theater in America
4. To read, discuss, and understand plays
5. To use computers and technology to enhance training
6. To create a final project (theatrical performance) for IEP students, staff, friends, and family

With English being a second language to all of these students, it is crucial to learn these skills. When the conceptual training has entered its threshold, the real training and practice comes from integrating drama activities. Some exercises that these students are assigned to include attending live plays and responding to assigned readings (Dodson, 2002). This allows the students to first observe, but then later participate and expand on the experience of both (Dodson, 2002). Furthermore, vocal warm-ups are a great way to begin a lesson (Dodson, 2002). Many of the students come from as many as five different language backgrounds (Dodson, 2002). Each particular student had different challenges that needed to be overcome (Dodson, 2002). However, overarching areas of improvement were articulation, volume, intonation, phrasing, and word groups (Dodson, 2002). Computers and technology were also used as learning aids. There was a website (http://www.colostate.edu/depts/writingCenter/ceilidh/ad440/forum.htm) that was used to provide students with additional computer-based training and a web forum for students to communicate and have active discussions on lessons that were learned (Dodson, 2002). This also allows students to write for their peers and not just teachers as they were normally used to (Dodson, 2002).

IMPROVISATION

One capability that assists in making SPs effective is the use of improvisation. According to Mike Napier, Improvisation is "getting on a stage and making stuff up as you go". Improvisation can be used heavily in comedy, and is partially used in SP training. SPs must be able to improvise. However, their improvisation must be held within the constraints of the scenario. Concepts of improvisation can be learned, but the best method to improve at it is to simply do it. There used to be a show called "Whose Line is it Anyways?", which consisted of three to four actors who simply were involved in improvisation. These techniques allow the actors to think quickly on their feet, and provide a quick-witted response.

Mike Napier discussed the rules to Improvisation in his book "Improvise: Scene from the Inside Out". Below are the rules:

1. **"Don't deny"**
2. **"Don't ask questions"**
3. **"Don't dictate action"**
4. **"Don't talk about past or future events"**
5. **"Establish who, what, where"**
6. **"Don't negotiate"**
7. **"Don't do teaching scenes"**
8. **"Show, don't tell"**
9. **"Say, yes, and then say and"**
10. **"Don't talk about what you are doing"**

Bad improvisation scenes have particular patterns that have been observed by some experts (Napier, 2004). A common flaw in improvisation is when one person in the enactment is creating a fantasy of what the scene should be and the other character would not accept the reality of it (Napier, 2004). Sometimes, when there are rules that are ingrained in an actor's mind, they are more conscious of it and this occasionally removes the spontaneity of the interaction (Napier, 2004).

Fear has been a big factor for people to come up with a response. For example, if a child breaks something at home, they need to think of an excuse to break the news to their parents. If a person is preparing for an interview, they must prepare in advance so they are ready for any questions that may be asked. In improvisation, this same methodology must be used, but with less preparation time. The time to come up with a response is in seconds. When a response is elicited, the actor has this short amount of time to stop and think what options there are for a response and then choose one that fits best to accommodate a good response.

The first step to improvisation is to do something (Napier, 2004). There are many people who have steps and a plan to do something, but never get around to executing (Napier, 2004). In improvisation, there is no choice. The only choice is to act on instinct. Doing something could start from taking an active role in the scene. This will capture the audience and allow the actor to play a particular role in the interaction. In SP education, there is usually just a patient and a doctor, and when the SP truly takes initiative of the SP role, they can empower the role to be a more realistic representation of a medical case.

Although SPs are limited to the case, there can be different ways to start the scene to make it more realistic. The line that is chosen must be a line that is still relevant, but also engages the preceptor to react and truly become engaged in the doctor/patient interaction (Napier, 2004).

As mentioned in the earlier passage about playing back interactions, it is also wise for actors to see how they performed in the improvisations (Napier, 2004). These observations can allow the actors to see which traits were held onto and which ones were intermittent. When good traits are held throughout each dramatization, it shows a clear consistency in improvisation (Napier, 2004). An example of a good trait is having a possession of what is created, like when Dorothy held on to the desire of going back to Kansas. Although many other obstacles were being faced by Dorothy in her interactions, she held on to her objective of going home (Napier, 2004). SPs must also have this mentality when role-playing a patient. For example, although an SP drinks, smokes and has heart disease and cancer in her family, the main reason they are in the doctor's office is that they have an aching pain in the middle of their stomach and if they were to rate the pain between one and ten, the pain would be an eight.

Some common problems in improvisation can be too much exposition, talking too much, justifying what they are improvising, pausing for longer periods of time, and bailing on a point of view (Napier, 2004). Many of these traits show a lack of commitment and risk taking with the part that is taken on. When more commitment is provided to the role, then the actor will use their versatility to be able to adjust to the role and be immersed in the environment and character.

8

INTERACTIVE ACTING

INTERACTIVE ACTING

The concept of interactive acting is to truly bring your audience to a participation in the experience. In an SP encounter, the audience could be the medical student who is reacting to the actor. Jeff Wirth, the author of "Interactive Acting", is one of the pioneers of this technique of improvisation and audience interaction. This book speaks of four different kinds of Interactive Theater. The first type of interactive theater is the environmental theater (Wirth, 1994). This type of environment is where the audience is actually part of the experience. They are part of the experience as they can be individual actors as well. These audience members all have a particular role in the experience to train one another along with the actual student. This application can be very useful when training a teacher how to teach a class. The instructor can practice teaching a class of students and each of the students can have varying factors that may match the average demographic of the area where the instructor will be whether the factors vary by race, sex, social status, etc. There are also several individual lessons that can be taught about making particular decisions, public speech training, interviewing for a job, social worker training, etc. There are also video game engines that can be integrated into the technology to provide a more immersive experience as well.

The second concept that Wirth discusses is "playback theater" where scenes can be played from the audience's experience. This gives an actor a significant idea of how a specific group reacts to the actor's improvisation and character in a scenario. The comedian Aziz Ansari has a very innovative and calculated method of how he renders his comedy sketches. He plays back the crowds cheers, laughter, and overall responses to his jokes. He categorizes his jokes in different genres. When he sees high peaks in volume and laughter, he knows that those are good jokes. There was a time where he said a joke and the audience gave a mediocre response, but then noticed that when he said the same joke and spinned in a circle, he saw a significant increased response of laughter in the crowd. From learning these new lessons when utilizing media technology, he was able to customize and improve his sketches to get better responses from the audiences.

A third concept that Jeff Wirth discusses is Forum Theater, which is also known as the Theater of the Oppressed. This concept was initially developed by Augusto Boal (Improv, 2011) which focuses on social awareness and of the environment that the actor is in. There are limitations on a person's abilities within the scope of the acting area, and it promotes the actors to be cognizant of it. The final concept, which is an original concept developed by Jeff Wirth, is theatrical freestyle. This is when the audience participates with the actors and is integrated into a complete creation.

VIDEO GAME VOICE ACTORS

Many video game actors come from various backgrounds. Holt talks about a video game actor in particular who started out as a telemarketer (2011). Although not as glamorous as it sounds, it allowed young Adam Harrington, who is now known in many well-known video games such as Rift, Test Drive Unlimited 2, League of Legends, 25 to Life and Puzzle Agents, to be creative in his job (Holt, 2011). To spice up his workday, he would begin speaking to some of his clients in an accent that was similar to the particular area that he was calling (Holt, 2011). One example of this was when New York fire fighters would call-in (Holt, 2011). He later took voice acting classes where he learned more than just accents but how to become a character (Holt, 2011). As mentioned before about the importance of mentoring, Adam was able to make a significant mentor out of his teacher Susan McCollom (Holt, 2011). He has built quite a broad skill set and versatility of voices ranging from African American characters to beach personalities, people from the south, and Arabic accents (Holt, 2011).

9

EXPERIENTIAL LEARNING

APPLYING AN EXPERIENTIAL PERSPECTIVE TO LEARNING

Experiential learning is the act of being able to learn a task or a skill set as you go, and the experiences that you develop grow and mature the more active practice that you have. Experiential learning can be beneficial especially in standardized patient training as the Standardized Patients can get up to speed on learning their lines for the SP case as they actively practice the case.

According to Baker, conversational learning provides a major training tool as learners can create new lessons learned as they experience new ones; and build new knowledge through their interactions.

10

MEDICAL FOCUS GROUPS

INSIGHT FROM PANEL MEMBERS

A Medical Expert Focus Group consisted of 3 Medical Doctors, a Director of SP Education at a College of Medicine, and two SP educators. The current way that SPs are trained at institutions is that they are emailed a medical case in advance. Upon receiving the medical case in advance, the SPs are expected to learn the case and then later have a discussion about it with the educators. After this, practice in role-playing is done, a dress rehearsal, and a dry run. Some of the less experienced SPs get more attention than the veteran SPs. An avatar that can bring an SP to proficiency would be an asset to the training along with providing the ability to have some extra training at home before the discussion with the educator.

SP RESPONSE DISCREPANCIES

A standard answer is expected from an SP, but often times the answer is not phrased exactly as scripted. To accommodate this, a guide is created to show acceptable answers that are within the acceptable range of answers. After this interaction is complete, a third person reviews the case and evaluates the communication skills. Something to consider is that medical students do not always ask questions in the same way or order as scripted. An example of this is if the medical student were to ask the SP if they take drugs. The question would need to be executed to specify if it was referring to illicit drugs or prescriptions. Another example is if the Medical Doctor were to ask an SP "Do you read?" The answer could either be if the SP was able to read or be completely illiterate. The SPs should not be over-trained to expect the questions in the same order as well to prevent them from being scripted. Both Avatars and Pre-recorded humans provide training value to SPs. The Avatar could be helpful to ask sensitive questions as some people feel more comfortable with an avatar as opposed to a human. However, this might pose a fidelity issue when having training time on a virtual human and then transferring to real humans. Although, SPs are now more tech savvy than before, which could provide a more accepted response.

DRAWBACKS AND SOLUTIONS

The drawbacks to having a Pre-recorded human are that the scripting is limited. If an avatar has an artificial intelligence system and natural language processing, it may be a better tool than Pre-recorded video delivery. The training effectiveness could be improved by examining how the SP performs during history taking. Behavioral responses are getting better now such as non-verbal cues, smiles, and nods that can be programmed. What would add to training effectiveness would be to have the avatars be plural instead of singular in a virtual world like Second Life. This virtual world could have a headshot of the individual who is being trained. This virtual world gives context to the training. The benefits to having avatars are that certain parts can be exaggerated on certain factors to pick up details so that distracting components are eliminated.

VIRTUAL HUMANS VS. VIDEO PLAYBACK IN SP TRAINING

One of the medical doctors mentioned that a comparison of the two depends on the case. In training medical students, a symptom which cannot be seen (headache, fever) would be good with a Pre-recorded Human, but a sign which a doctors can see (trauma, swelling) would be best expressed with a Virtual Human. There was one case where an SP had a dislocated shoulder and the SP had to maintain a posture to simulate this. Something like this would have been a good approach with two solutions side by side. The benefits vary depending on the task. The benefits for each of the medical cases also vary depending on the learning style of the SP. Some SPs learn cognitively, while others learn more visually or physically. If there is a high fidelity in robots, there is a large training value in integrating this technology in cross-training. One of the most important tasks in SP training is history taking. History taking probably amounts to about 30% of the interview, while the physical exam represents 40%. The remaining 30% involves advising of the patient, treatment, and counseling. At this point it cannot be predicted how SP training evolves, but it would be beneficial to also add trauma and post-op to some of the training of cases. In addition, the test, evaluation, and curriculum may have more stringent requirements in the future. Subject matter experts and healthcare professionals should also be leveraged heavily to verify the validity of the cases and content. Both Avatars and pre-recorded humans are good tools, but together are powerful. One of the most important drivers is which provides the cheapest solution short-term and long-term.

OPEN ENDED FEEDBACK FROM MEDICAL STUDENTS WHO TOOK THE STEP 2 CS

Below is some open ended feedback that was given from some medical students that experienced an interaction with an SP, when taking their Step 2 CS board exam.

Medical Student#1: "The Step 2 CS was pretty easy. The SPs didn't really re-act the scenarios pretty well. I wish they had some type of simulation for me to practice doing interviews with different cases in a simulation for the board exam".

Medical Student#2: "The SPs acted very poorly when trying to portray a case, and I was just trying to get the exam over with. It's kind of a hassle, because sometimes you have to go out of state to take the exam. I wish they had it via teleconference or could get credit through some kind of simulation as the test is pretty expensive as well".

Medical Student#3 "The SPs are horrible actors. When they cough, they don't sound like they are really coughing, and the expression on their face doesn't seem convincing enough to believe that they are really sick. Sometimes, they give the answer away if you don't understand how they feel, which could give an unfair advantage".

Medical Student#4 "The SPs are very robotic, and they didn't seem realistic at all in the case that they portrayed".

Medical Student#5 "The Step 2 CS is not really a big deal if you pass, but it is a HUGE deal if you fail it, because it affects if you get into a good residency program. Sometimes the SPs give the answer away with the way they act, and if they feel a connection with the student, they might have a bias which could lead to an unfair advantage".

Medical Student #6 "My Step 2 CS exam went fine. The SPs that I had were really good actors, and they portrayed the case very well. However, I did take the test in LA, and am not sure if the location plays a big role in the quality of SPs. Most people in the LA/Hollywood area are trained actors on the side. But at the same time, I was very nervous about the test and might have thought the SP was a good actor either way as I was just trying to pass the exam".

11

VIRTUAL HUMANS AND SIMULATION SUMMARY

SUMMARIZING EMBODIED CONVERSATIONAL AGENTS AND THEIR EDUCATIONAL APPLICATIONS

In the research above, it can be seen that ECAs can provide a benefit when it comes to interfacing with virtual environments and acting as educational agents, mentors, and role-players. According to Bailenson, humans feel more comfortable with avatar actors in embarrassing situations than they do with actors (2005). In addition, some of the pressure is relieved when being cognizant of the fact that they are interfacing with an agent that is similar to a human-like character. This is one of the discoveries that we realize when dealing with some subjects who are interfacing with an avatar and some that are not.

VIRTUAL HUMANS AND THEIR ADDED LEVEL OF COMFORT

The VHs provide a sense of detachment from real life which can increase the level in comfort although having a lower sense of presence (Conkey, 2010). This is important because prominent research has indicated that higher presence equates to more involvement and participation for a better training tool (Conkey, 2010). The study performed by Curtis

Conkey which compared machinima training with video content delivery for soft skills training showed no change in the results. This means that the avatar based machinima had no difference in results than the training tool that had recorded human actors. What does this mean? It shows that a virtual human-based tool for training applications can provide a contribution to the medical community that is just as effective as a pre-recorded human version. Furthermore, this alternative provides more reuse, customization, briefing, debriefing, ethnic diversity in training, and an ability to update capability.

THE RESEARCH EXPEDITION

The objective of this research expedition is to see if change can be seen when applying these aspects to a Standardized Patient Training tool which compares Virtual Humans to Pre-Recorded Humans. Below is the list of assumptions that were gathered from the primary objectives:

Assumption 1:

Training SPs with experiential learning can reduce some time that SPs need to train on in a real simulated examining room for learning the task of knowledge transfer of a basic non-physical exam.

Assumption 2:

Using Virtual humans in training does not provide an immediate cost savings up front as there are detailed developmental efforts needed to create the layers for the intelligence that is needed for the ECAs. However, over time, there would be some savings in faculty time; resources, time to train, and possibly one day replace the need for live standardized patients in medical board exams.

Assumption 3:

Embodied conversational agents can simulate gestures, facial displays, and emotion that can provide communication skills training to help SPs (actors) possibly learn their lines/medical case/rating abilities in a shorter time frame. Thus, as mentioned, this could assist in reducing time and resources in the examining room.

12 FUTURE APPROACHES IN EDUCATION AND TECHNOLOGY

NATURAL LANGUAGE PROCESSING

The advancements in natural language processing have developed slowly, but the challenges still exist in fidelity, speech understanding, speech recognition, and lag in processing time of messages. The Roleplay trainer could later be integrated with the Interpersonal Simulator to accommodate standardized patient training with artificial intelligence, voice recognition, and voice understanding.

CODING FOR INTERRATER RELIABILITY

An SP and SME could be required to complete a checklist to rate the medical student to teach medical student evaluation skills. The SP will complete this immediately after the role-playing exercise, and the SME will do this at a later convenient time. The role-playing performance exercise will be recorded, archived, and reviewed for coding by the SME. The SMEs will also be watching the archived video to rate how well the SP performed on the standardized patient encounter. In conclusion, the measures from the checklists will be a rater checklist from the SP and SME and the differences can be seen in results between the SP and SME responses in the checklists.

USING REAL SPS

A study could be done with real SPs to show the learning transfer that a true application can be seen. Furthermore, if these studies prove to show benefit to the SPs, then the Roleplay Trainer could implement the Interpersonal Simulator to provide conversationally modeled standardized medical students for SP training.

AUTOMATED ASSESSMENTS

Finding ways for avatars to automatically assess the SP in conjunction to the training exercise can also provide value and reduction in unnecessary staffing.

RECRUITING SPS FROM BROADWAY AND HOLLYWOOD

In big cities like New York and Los Angeles, actors play significant roles, like a woman named Quinn Lemly who plays a character that is staged in a 1940s theme where sparkling evening gowns are the center of attention (Lagnado, 2011). However, on some days that Quinn is not auditioning or performing, she will be on her way to the Weill Cornell Medical College to act as an SP (Lagnado, 2011). Some of these standardized patient opportunities can pay up to $25 dollars an hour (Lagnado, 2011). The Weill Cornell Medical College in Manhattan is fully equipped with medical examining rooms that provide full capabilities for SPs to see where they made mistakes, see how it should be done, and provide two-way mirrors for faculty to see the interactions (Lagnado, 2011).

With the current economy, the SP programs lead by Dr. Kang in New York and Denise Lock from the University of Southern California's Keck's School of Medicine have seen a significant increase in actors looking for opportunities (Lagnado, 2011). Keck's medical program has hired individuals with acting experience in television shows and other commercials (Lagnado, 2011). Some portrayals that actors have performed are heart attacks, diabetes, Parkinson's, and hot flashes (Lagnado, 2011). The only issue is that sometimes the actors want the take things to an area that is out of scope of the scenario (Lagnado, 2011). However casting of these

SPs can be difficult at times as Dr. Kang mentions "we want stars but we need to temper their star quality" (Lagnado, 2011). Some features that could be added in simulation to allow further applications to train acting would be to have more realistic facial expressions in avatars, and provide the ability to point to where the pain is.

SIXTH SENSE TECHNOLOGY

Gestures are used for everyday emotions and expressions of different types of messages (Mistry, 2009). Some gestures are so common that they are assumed to have a meaning (Mistry, 2009). For example, a shrugging of shoulders might mean that a person is indifferent, or pointing at something might indicate a certain direction that must be approached (Mistry, 2009). These gestures can now be used as a human machine interface with the help of Pranav Mistry's Sixth Sense technology (Mistry, 2009) Such gestures like moving a page as done on the iPad, pinching an image to expand its dimensions, or even joining two thumbs and index fingers while forming a rectangle to take a picture are effective in initiating commands (Mistry, 2009). This concept is to not limit the information gathering of the information age to only the mobile realm, but to leverage off of the mobile technology's bandwidth to allow humans to interact with their biological surroundings, thus making any wall a touch screen and making any piece of paper a tablet (Mistry, 2009). Thus, the digital world can be taken with the individual (Mistry, 2009). Using this technology into the immersive world assists in simulating a physical interview, where a standardized patient can be touched by a doctor for certain signs and symptoms.

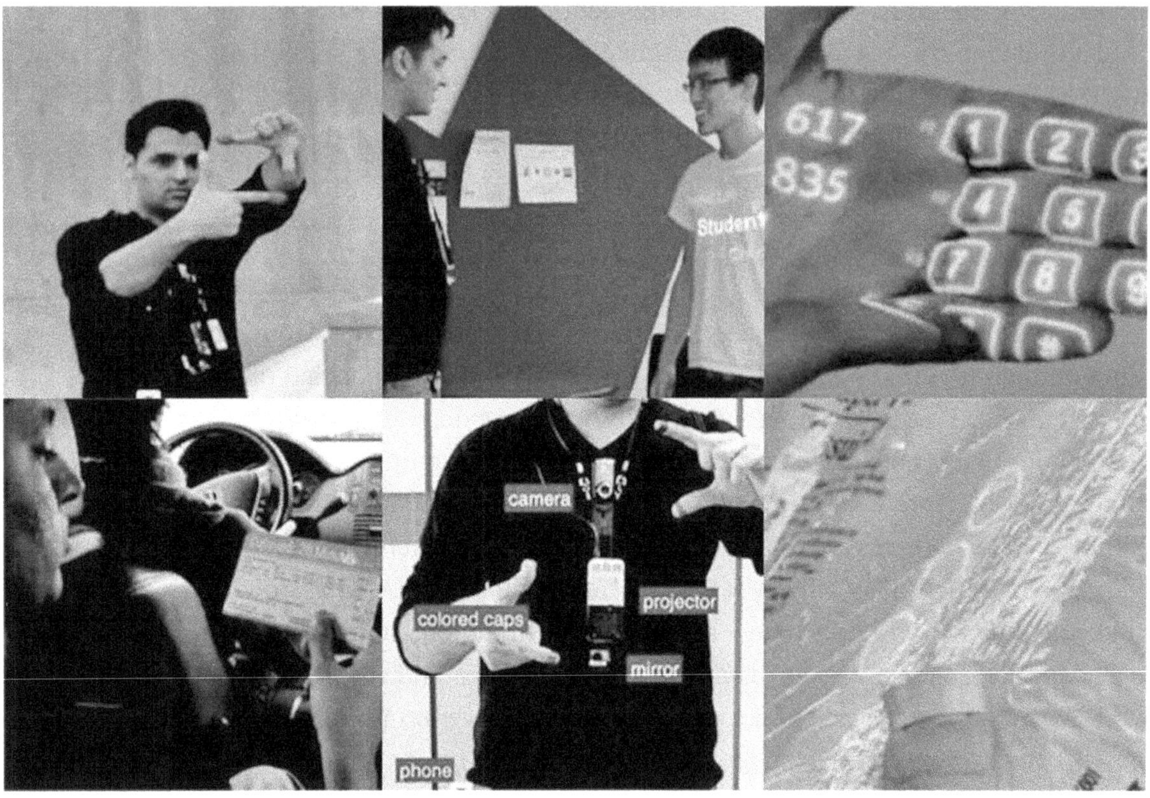

Figure 5: Sixth Sense Technology

(Permission to use image granted by Pranav Mistry)

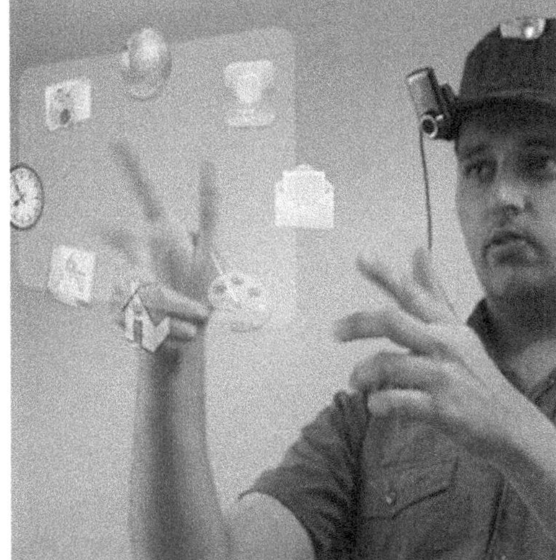

Figure 6: Sixth Sense Virtual Tablet PC

(Permission to use image granted by Pranav Mistry)

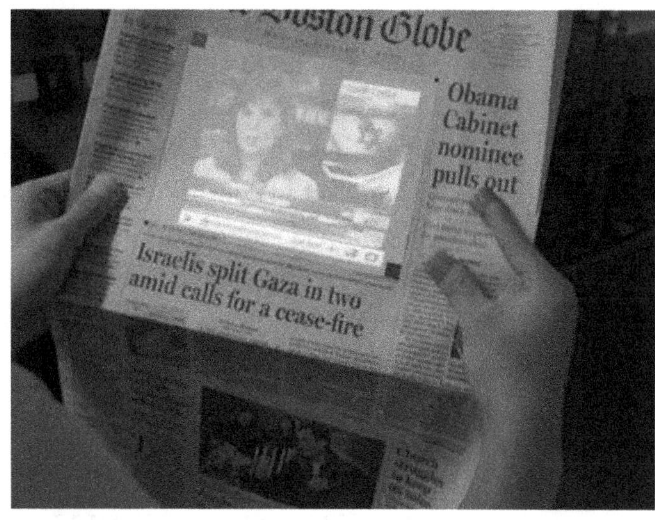

Figure 7: Sixth Sense Technology: Projection of Feeds

(Permission to use of image granted by Pranav Mistry)

When seeing this technology, it can be observed that the technology that is currently being developed is not too far from what is seen in the movies (Mistry, 2009). A similar human machine interface was one that was portrayed in the movie “Minority Report”.

HOLOGRAMS AND HOLOMERS

Holograms are a popular technology that brings an added dimension to the realism that is desired in the entertainment industry. Now this technology is being leveraged for several military and medical applications. A briefing that was presented by M. Beth H. Pettit in the year 2009 to discuss the research plans for the joint medical simulation technology showed relevance to using holograms for training anatomy (Pettit, 2009). This could be useful in standardized patient education when dealing with cases that are related to post-operation. Later, a Request for Information (RFI) was issued by the United States Army that reached out to public companies and industry to produce a viable technical solution that provides three dimensional (3-D) holographic imaging (US Army, 2010). These images are required to be functional without the need of 3-D glasses (US Army, 2010). The overall mission and desires are to improve the quality of training that exists and allow better technology to bring troops to a higher level of competency in medical specialties (US Army, 2010).

On the other hand, Holomers (Holographic Medical Electronic Representation) are complete scans of an individual's body (Virtual, 2011). These graphical representations can be used to help understand the body and realize preventative measures that can be developed to provide a better understanding of the physiological conditions. By taking blood and saliva samples, the biological information can eventually be integrated with the physical model and provide an opportunity for a three dimensional medical record. There will be a time where every patient will have their own distinct holomer (Virtual, 2011). If a complex surgical procedure needs to be performed on a patient, the planning, preparation, and practice can be done on this digital representation (Virtual, 2011).

STRETCHING VISUAL IMAGES TO REDUCE PAIN

A psychological test was completed to see if the stretching of visual images of a body could affect tolerance to certain types of pain (Mancini, 2011). When a subject was given an amount of heat to their hand, the pain was tolerable when the hand was seen on a reflection where the hand was stretched to seem larger than it was (Mancini, 2011). Two lessons can be gathered from this. One is that when we see some body parts being stretched, it allows in some areas to be more tolerable to pain (Mancini, 2011). Second, when the hands were out of sight, the pain was less tolerable, so it can be concluded that the hands must be seen to endure a larger tolerance.

SIMILARITY EFFECTS TO TEACHING

In a study that was performed by some researchers, a total of 257 subjects were involved in a study that involved a training in Excel, where different questions were asked by an avatar (Behrend, 2011). The similar looks of the trainer had less of an impact than the subjective inclination to the educator (Behrend, 2011). The subjective feedback was compared with the objective feedback and this study proves that projections on how the training will perform could be better visualized when utilizing a subjective format (Behrend, 2011). Subjects provided inputs on how much they liked the trainer (Behrend, 2011). The avatar seemed to be most engaging when it had similar characteristics and representations of the user, and possessed similar teaching styles (Behrend, 2011). When training standardized patients, the applications of avatars that have a closer relevance to the user might provide a more powerful training tool.

USING ARTIFICIAL INTELLIGENCE FOR RESOLVING DISPUTES

According to an article in the "Wall Street Journal", GE is using a technology to handle resolutions that are relevant to disputes in the oil and gas sectors (O'Connell, 2011). This software handles the bidding process and works to come to a settlement (O'Connell, 2011). The software is managed by an engineer, and will provide cost savings in legal fees and personnel (O'Connell, 2011). Although this system was criticized for not having a human element, if effective it could be beneficial to the energy arena (O'Connell, 2011). Similarly in medical simulation, if avatars prove to be just as effective as they were in this study, there is potential for cost savings and process optimization when viable logic in medical decisions is displayed.

INTEGRATING MOBILE TECHNOLOGY INTO STANDARDIZED PATIENT EDUCATION

Mobile Technology is growing and not going away. These technological instruments are becoming miniature computers that will be the next generation for education, transactions, and technology development. Although there can be security threats, there are also significant benefits to mobile learning with the new smart phone technology that is available. David Metcalf delivered an interested keynote address in 2006 regarding learning for the mobile society. Based on data, blended learning that is integrated in the flow of particular processes can provide a framework to provide information at the essential time that it is needed (Metcalf, 2006). One type of education could be delivered one time, but in different formats (Metcalf, 2006). The phones could not only be used two ways as people primarily use them; but the people and the systems, and the systems of systems have allowed certain processes to be simpler. "In the field, in your hands, on demand" and "stolen moments of learning" are quotes that Dr. Metcalf uses at the keynote address. This allows us to maximize productivity in how we deliver learning, and learn through doing (Metcalf, 2006). He was able to write his book through his spare time using a special pen that transcribes text. Being able to have a holistic blended learning solution can allow the ability to improve processes.

PODCASTING AND PUBLISHING TO GET THE RIGHT INFORMATION AT THE RIGHT TIME

A new trend alongside blogs is podcasting. This allows the ability to be able to subscribe to feeds that can be setup from the phone. In addition to subscribing, podcasts can be created and shared to social media sites from websites like www.podbean.com. These podcasts can also be recorded from a phone and published with websites like www.audioblog.com, www.asterisk.org, www.garageband.com, and www.gabcast.com (Metcalf, 2006). Educators can keep their courses fresh and in real time by software that allows to provide content that publishes content onto websites (Metcalf, 2006).

Advanced technologies of location awareness will eventually be able to allow people to pass by someone and receive information that could potentially have areas of interest that another might possess. This ability to share expert information can provide information from ebooks, audiofiles, and videos can also provide information at the right time (Metcalf, 2006). These multiple modalities could provide to be effective if applied for the right use (Metcalf, 2006). This could provide great opportunities for technological collaboration and return on investment (Metcalf, 2006).

Understanding these technologies and how they can be used to assist in clinical skills education can provide awareness on how performance needs can be met (Metcalf, 2006).

TECHNOLOGICAL SINGULARITY

The concept of Technological Singularity most popularized by many futurists such as Ray Kurzweil and Vernor Vinge is the hypothesis that technology will reach a phase where it might potentially intersect the intelligence of that of a human being (Technological Singularity, 2012). This intelligence could potentially surpass that of a humans through technological interchange (Technological Singularity, 2012). Kurzweil believes that this is due to paradigm shifts in technology and Moore's Law (Technological Singularity, 2012). This exponential growth in computing power is the cause of this especially in the areas of speed and intelligence (Technological Singularity, 2012). The implications and precautions that are necessary should be taken to ensure that the impact to humanity causes no harm (Technological Singularity, 2012). Isaac Asimov lists three laws that govern the guidelines for robotics: "(1) A robot may not injure a human being or, through inaction, allow a human being to come to harm", "(2) A robot must obey orders given to it by human beings except where such orders would conflict with the First Law", and "(3) A robot must protect its own existence as long as such protection does not conflict with either the First or Second Law (Technological Singularity, 2012)." When reading about the temperament of a puppy at an adoption agency, some breeds are pack leaders. However, the master should never allow the puppy to be the pack leader of a family. Similarly, even when technological singularity is achieved, the humans should still be the pack leader and the robots should still be seen as machines that are created to perform tasks to assist in the quality of living and performance of human beings.

INTEGRATING MIXED REALITY AND SURGICAL SIMULATION FOR SP APPLICATIONS

Most Standardized Patients are used for simple physical exams or non-physical exams. These skill sets that can often be in-depth from a surgical perspective should also be trained on with SPs. But the recurring issue is that the SPs don't truly have the symptoms, trauma, or wounds as they are healthy actors. Thus, good surgical training cannot be trained on an SP. This surgical integration will then leverage off of the use of simulation. The military now has rubber suits made of synthetic skin that an actor or role-playing soldier can wear to simulate trauma in the battlefield. This suit will actually bleed if you cut it. If you cut deep enough it will include simulated body parts, which actually have smells of urine and blood. These fluids can be fabricated through advanced materials laboratories and provide a special level of fidelity that cannot normally be provided with mannequins. Another example of more elaborate exams is when using virtual humans for exams in more private areas of the body and/or sensitive clinical skills interviews. The standardized patients can also train with virtual doctors in an immersive environment for mixed reality physical exams (Kotranza, 2008). Some of these systems provide feedback to where the virtual human can be conversationally modeled with a personality so that the modeled

personality can provide reactions within the real world as an expression of the virtual human or conversational model (Kotranza, 2008).

The Surgical Robot, also known as the Da Vinci system created by the company Intuitive, provides several benefits to surgery, but one of the largest benefits is that the system is not only easier on the patient, but it is easier on the doctor. These units have been popular for hysterectomies and prostatectomy procedures. However, these machines are quite expensive, and would require a great deal of resources, to be up and running simply for training. The solution is providing a simulated environment where they can train and first learn simple laparoscopic and surgical skills, and then be able to train on a simulated procedure until they have a very low error rate. Below are examples of surgical simulations and trainers provided by Mimic Technologies that allows for these types of training.

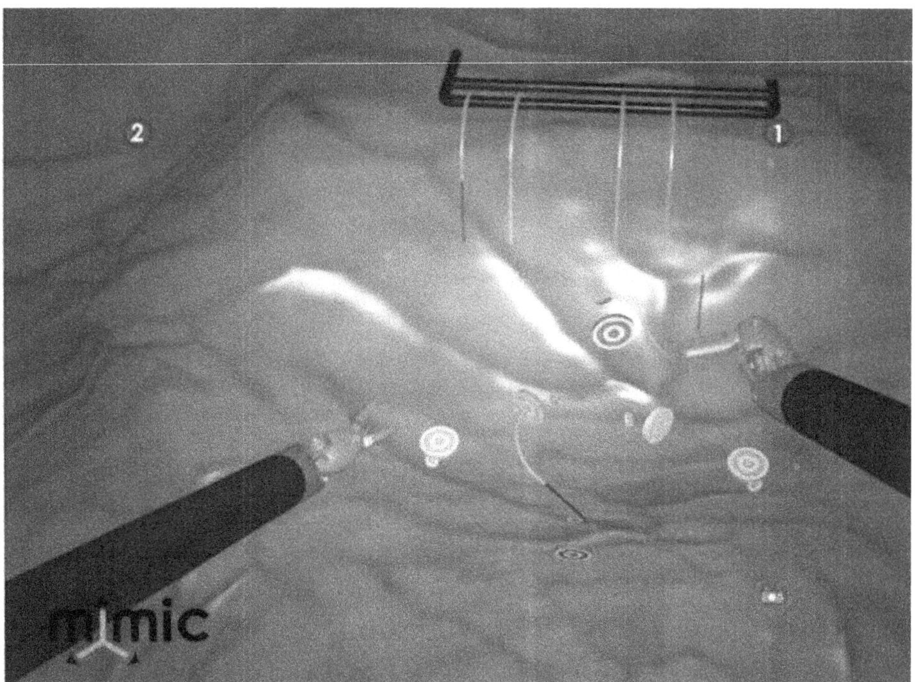

Figure 8: Needle Targeting Using MIMIC's Robotic Surgery Simulation

Permission to use image granted by MIMIC Technologies. Images can be retrieved at http://www.mimicsimulation.com/company/images-resources.php

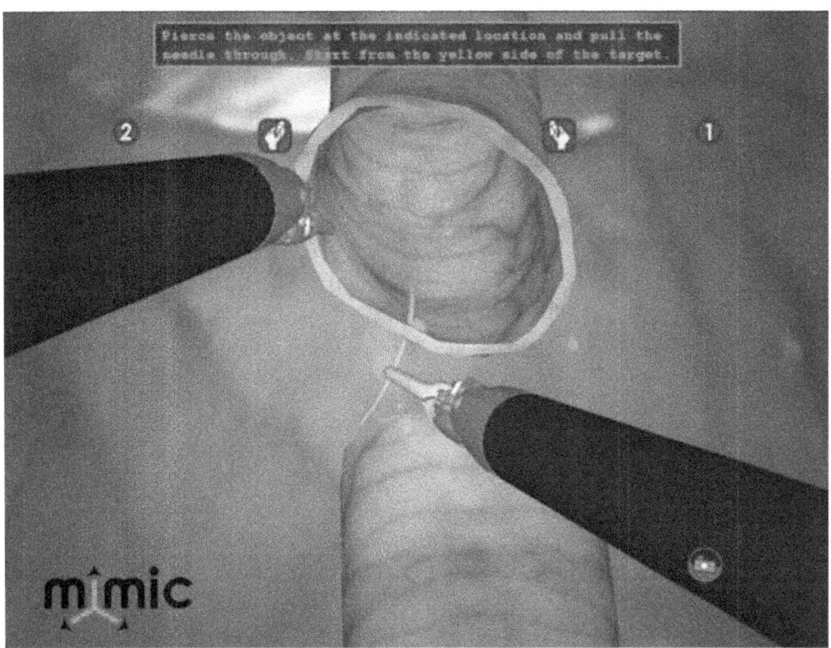

Figure 9: Pulling a Needle Through Tubes

Permission to use image granted by MIMIC Technologies. Images can be retrieved at http://www.mimicsimulation.com/company/images-resources.php

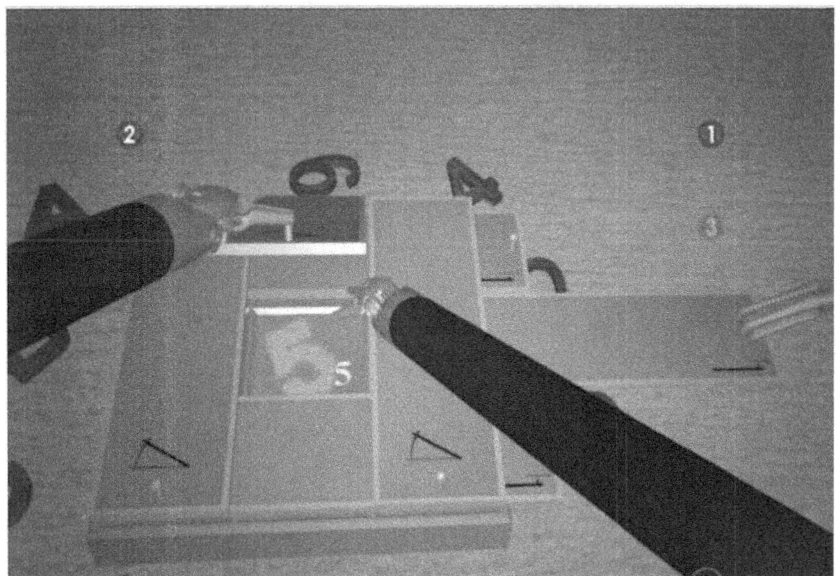

Figure 10: Matchboard

Permission to use image wgranted by MIMIC Technologies. Images can be retrieved at http://www.mimicsimulation.com/company/images-resources.php

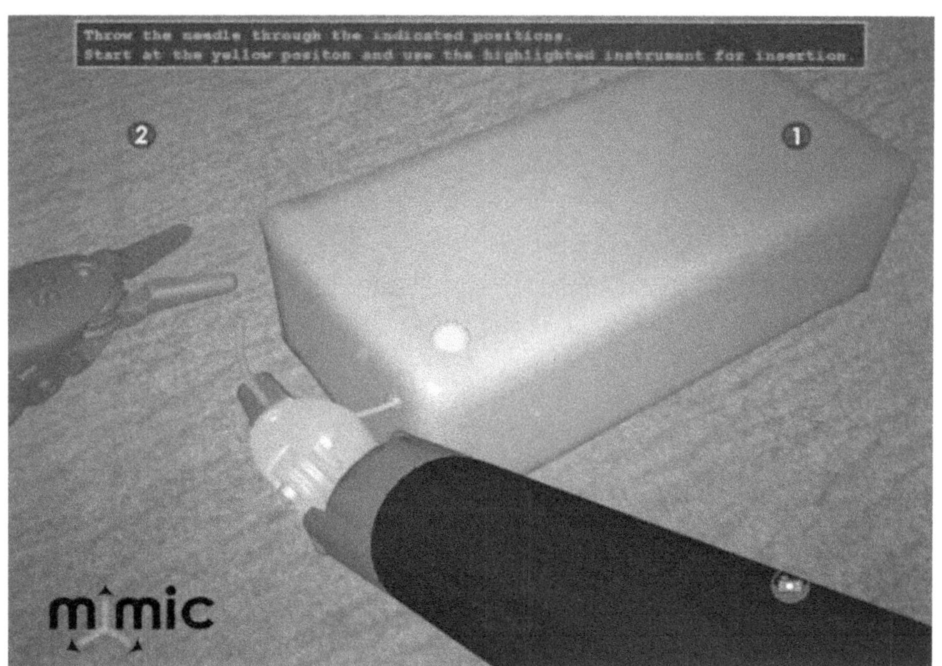

Figure 11: Suture Sponge

Permission to use image granted by MIMIC Technologies. Images can be retrieved at http://www.mimicsimulation.com/company/images-resources.php

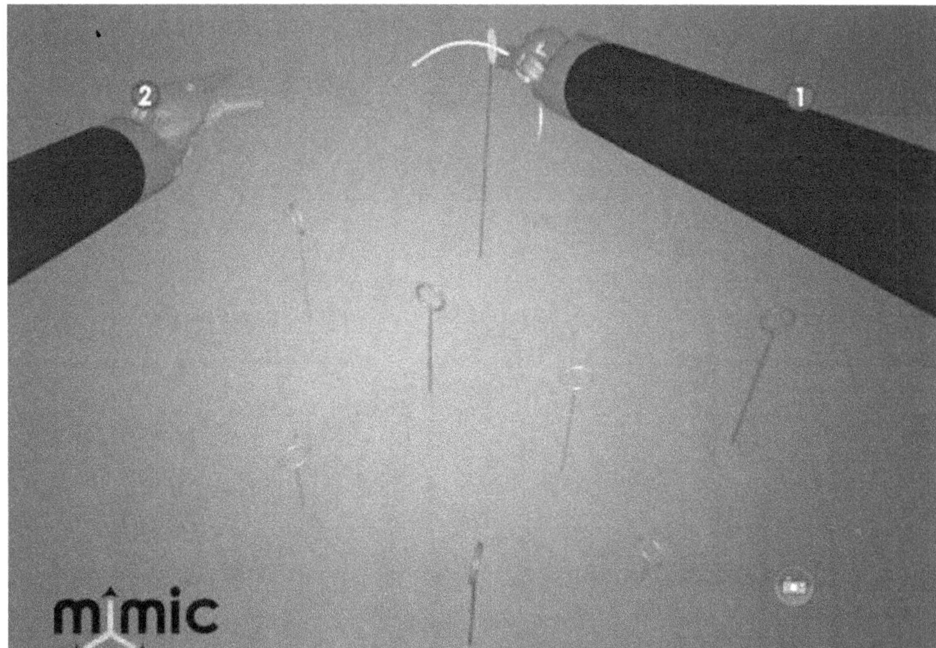

Figure 12: Thread and Rings

Permission to use image granted by MIMIC Technologies. Images can be retrieved at http://www.mimicsimulation.com/company/images-resources.php

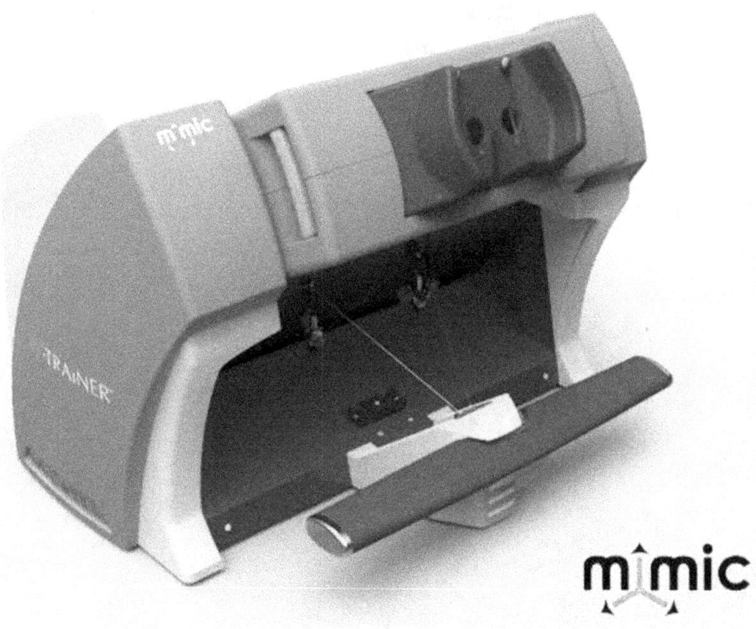

Figure 13: Da Vinci Trainer

Permission to use image granted by MIMIC Technologies. Images can be retrieved at http://www.mimicsimulation.com/company/images-resources.php

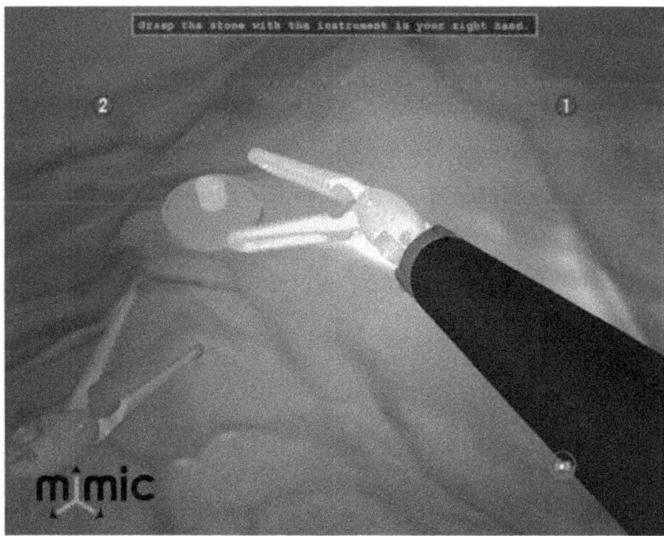

Figure 14: Camera Targeting

Permission to use image granted by MIMIC Technologies. Images can be retrieved at http://www.mimicsimulation.com/company/images-resources.php

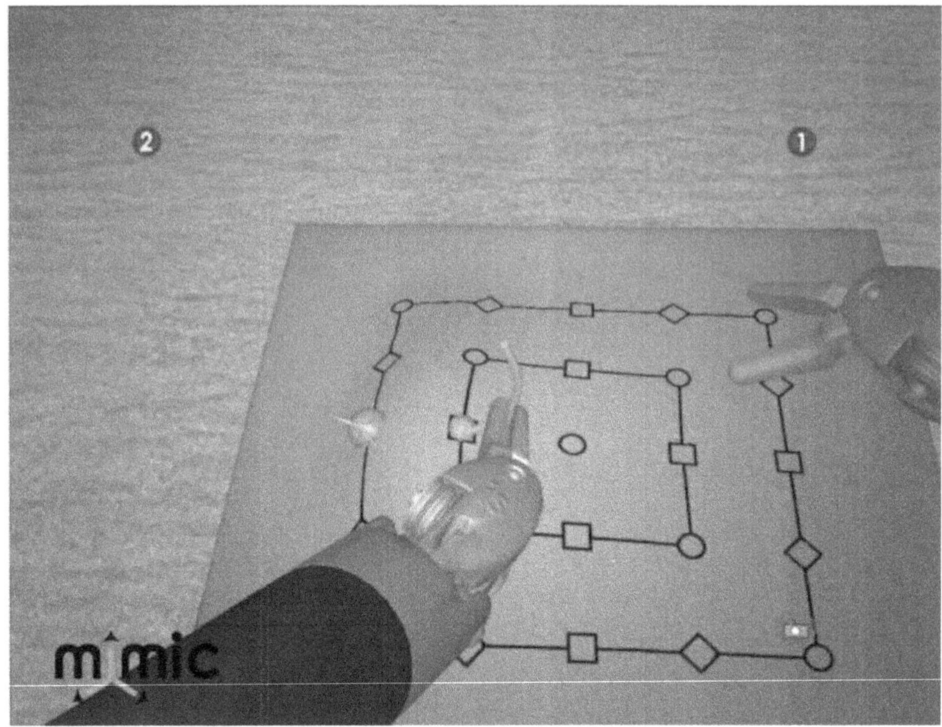

Figure 15: Dots and Needles

Permission to use image granted by MIMIC Technologies. Images can be retrieved at http://www.mimicsimulation.com/company/images-resources.php

On the following pages are some rich graphics provided by Biodigital Systems. Biodigital systems specialized in developing content for several applications in medical visualization. These images can be generated with the biodigital human tool at www.biodigitalhuman.com.

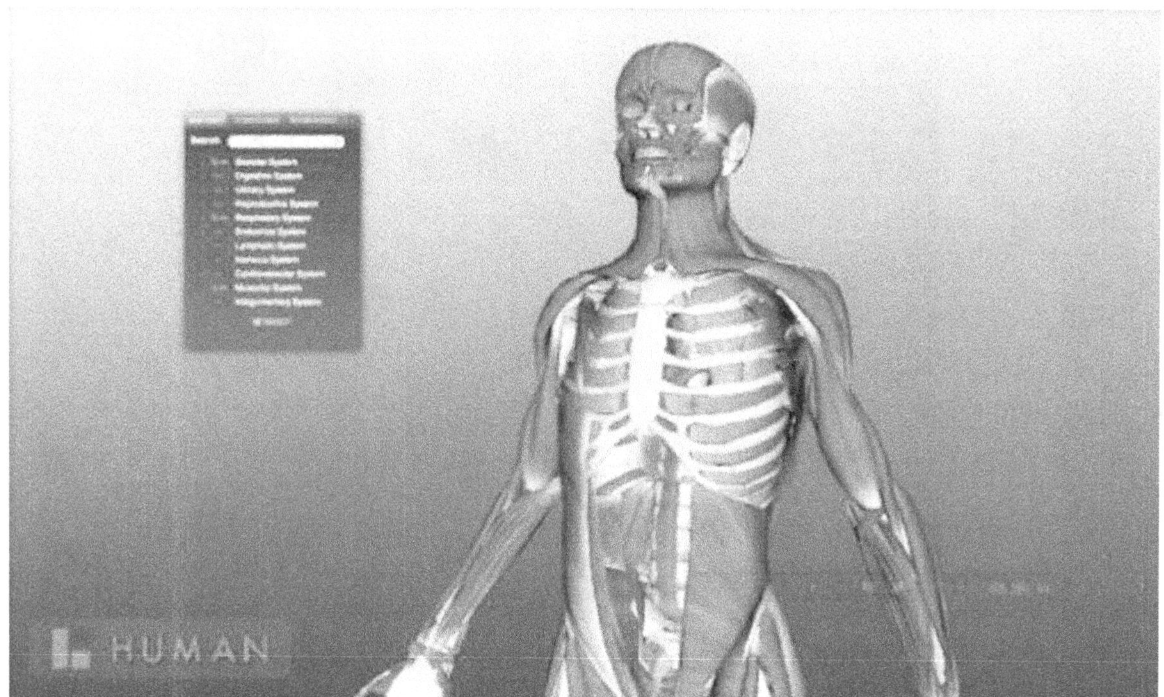

Figure 16: Biodigital Human 1

Permission to use image granted by Biodigital Systems screen capture
www.biodigitalhuman.com

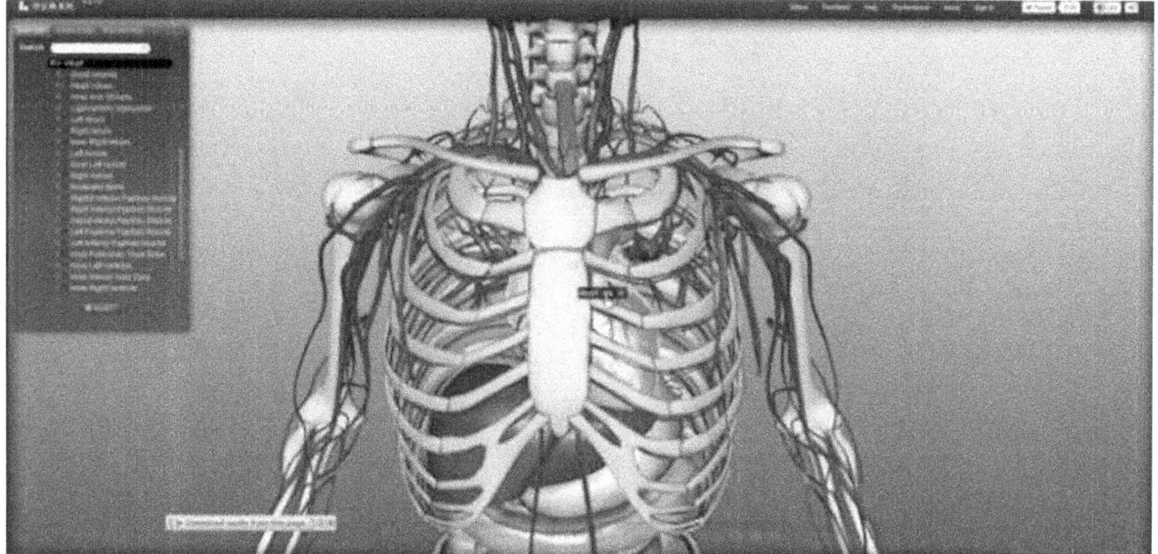

Figure 17: Biodigital Human 2

Permission to use image granted by Biodigital Systems screen capture
wwww.biodigitalhuman.com

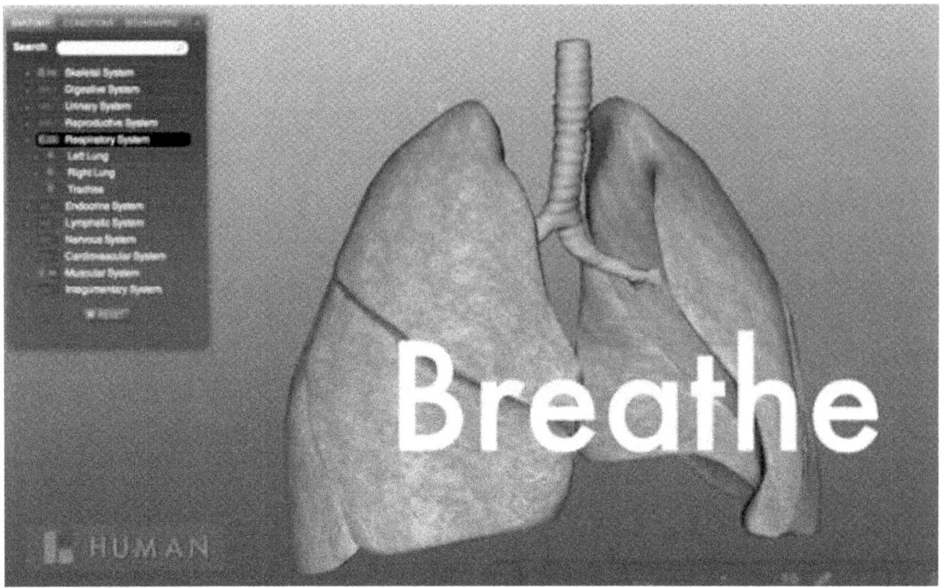

Figure 18: Lungs Animation

Permission to use image granted by Biodigital Systems screen capture www.biodigitalhuman.com

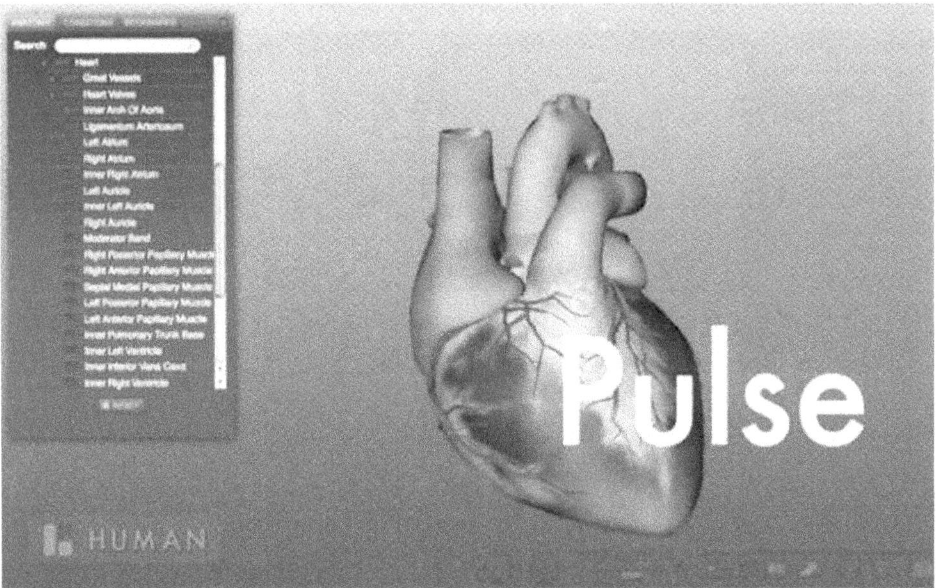

Figure 19: Heart Animation

Permission to use image granted by Biodigital Systems screen capture www.biodigitalhuman.com

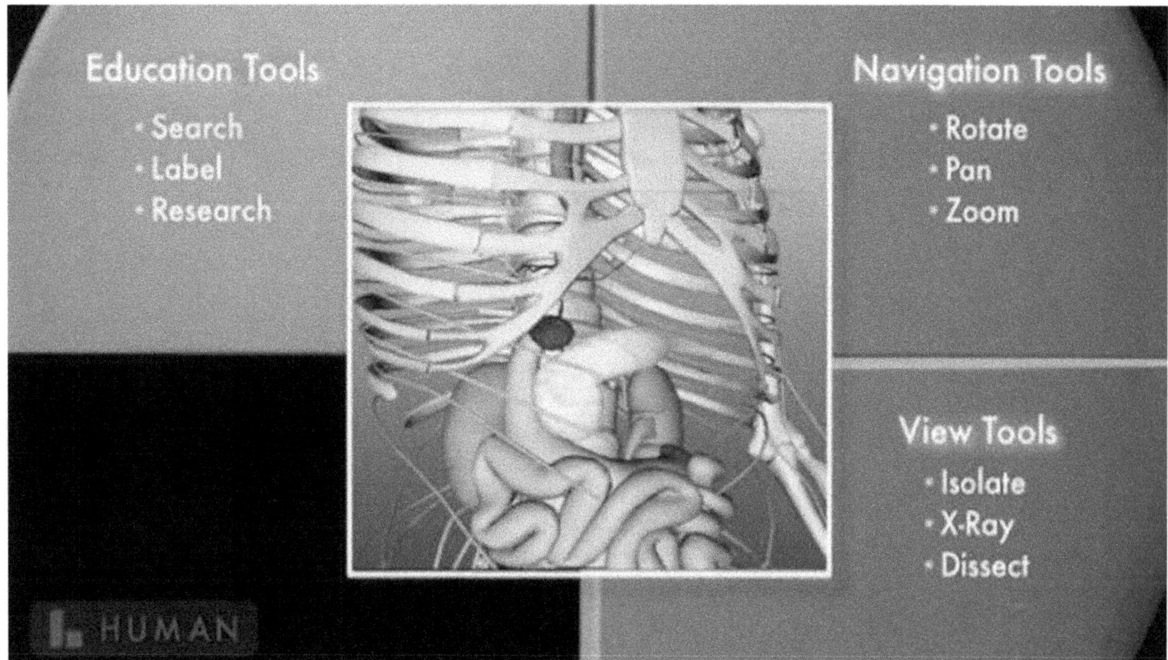

Figure 20: Educational, Navigation, and View Tools

Permission to use image granted by Biodigital Systems screen capture www.biodigitalhuman.com

APPENDIX A
ADDITIONAL DATA/ ARTIFACTS

The demographic data is utilized to understand if there are any significant differences among the demographic parameters. The Multiple ANOVA is conducted to analyze demographics.

Analysis of Variance for Assessment score, using Adjusted SS for Tests

Source	DF	Seq SS	Adj SS	Adj MS	F	P
Training method	1	1.923	1.057	1.057	0.11	0.745
Gender	1	40.297	11.675	11.675	1.18	0.283
Age	2	21.717	33.579	16.789	1.70	0.195
Race	4	129.068	116.032	29.008	2.94	0.032
Advanced degree (Yes/No)	1	1.063	3.863	3.863	0.39	0.535
Acting Experience (Yes/No)	1	1.442	1.317	1.317	0.13	0.717
Healthcare experience (Yes/No)	1	23.002	25.805	25.805	2.62	0.114
Bilingual (Yes/No)	1	6.735	6.735	6.735	0.68	0.414
Error	39	384.523	384.523	9.860		
Total	51	609.769				

The multiple ANOVA suggests that only "Race" is the significant factor indicating that at least one Race is different than others. In our study, there are five different Race types as Caucasian, Asian, Hispanic, African American, and Native American. But we do not know from ANOVA which Race different than other Races. To conduct this analysis, we conducted Tukey's test. The output is shown below.

Tukey 95% Simultaneous Confidence Intervals. All Pairwise Comparisons among Levels of Race. Individual confidence level = 99.33%

```
an subtracted from:

        Lower  Center   Upper
erican -2.580   2.250   7.080
        0.142   4.192   8.243
        0.461   5.000   9.539
rican  -1.660   8.000  17.660

        ----+---------+---------+---------+---

erican            (----+----)
                     (---+---)
                     (----+----)
rican              (--------+--------)
        ----+---------+---------+---------+---

          -10         0        10        20
```

```
Race = African American subtracted from:

Race                Lower  Center   Upper
Caucasian          -1.673   1.942   5.558
Hispanic           -1.406   2.750   6.906
Native American    -3.736   5.750  15.236

Race               ----+---------+---------+----
----+----

Caucasian                      (---+---)
Hispanic                        (---+---)
Native American              (--------+--------
)
                   ----+---------+---------+----
----+----

                     -10         0        10
20
```

Table 7: Additional Tukey Analysis

Charts of Pre and Post survey (For PANAS scale)

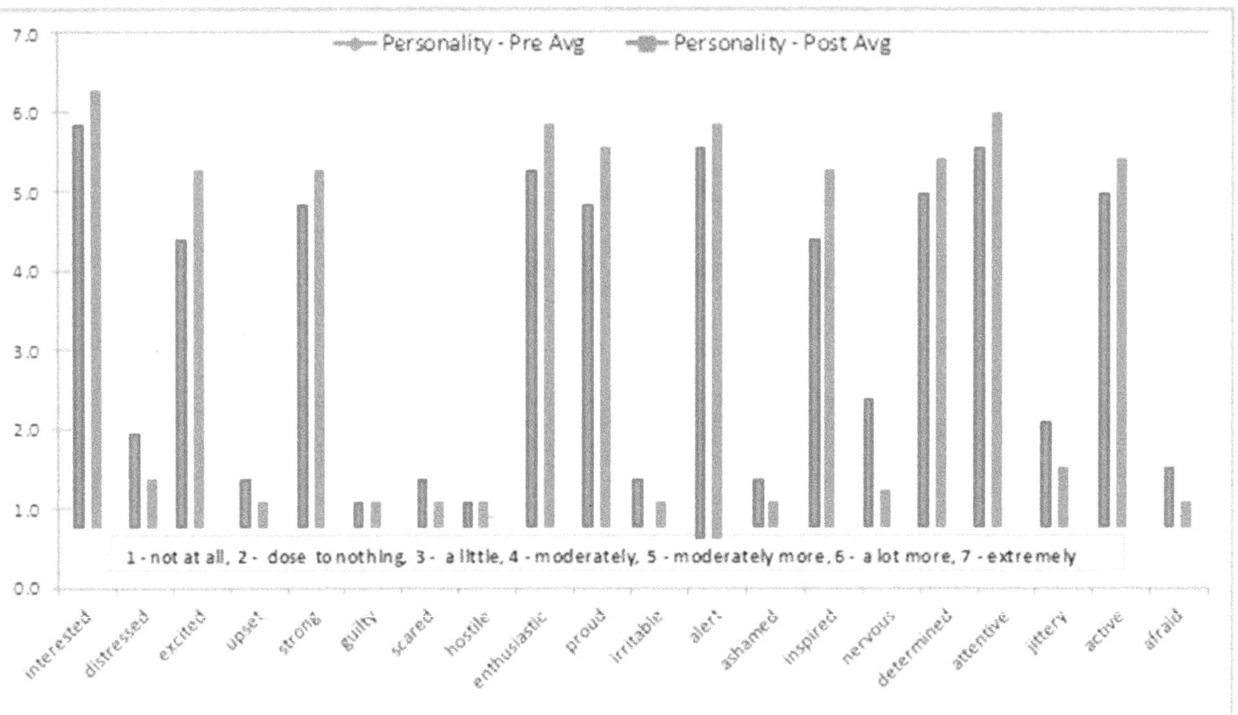

Table 8: Pre and Post Survey PANAS scales

The chart shows the subject's feeling at the present time using a PANAS (Positive and Negative Affect Schedule) scale before and after the study participation. The characteristics are on horizontal axis (X axis) and score (between 1 to 7) is on the vertical axis. The data showed positive movement for each category in the post survey. For example, subjects are more interested after the study, and subjects are less distressed after the study.

Chart of Perceived Usefulness Survey

The chart for perceived usefulness is plotted below. The description is assigned acronyms as shown below.

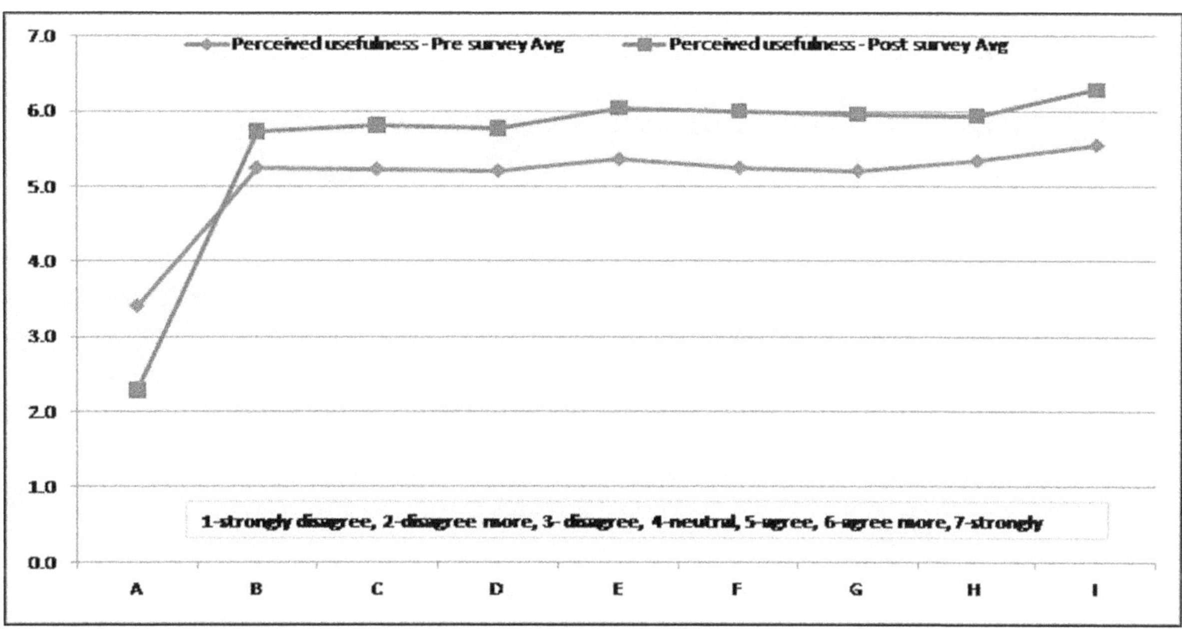

Table 9: Perceived Usefulness

DESCRIPTION	KEY
Training would be difficult to complete without computer based performance assessments	A
Using computer based performance assessments gives me more control of my training	B
Using computer based performance assessments improves my performance	C
Using computer based performance assessments addresses my training needs	D
Using computer based performance assessments saves me time	E
Using computer based performance assessments allows me to complete my tasks more quickly	F
Using computer based performance assessments enhances my effectiveness	G
Using computer based performance assessments makes it easier to learn	H
Overall, I find computer based performance assessments to be useful in learning	I

The data in the figure shows an overall positive attitude towards computer based performance assessments.

Chart for Perceived ease of use

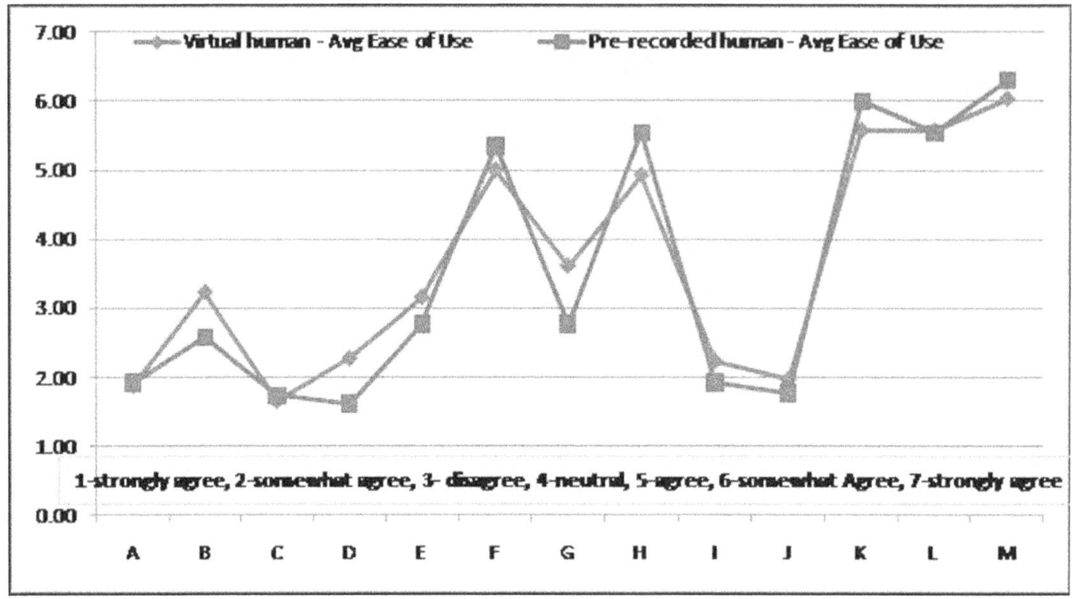

Table 10: Perceived Ease of Use

DESCRIPTION	KEY
I often get confused when I use computer based performance assessments	A
I make errors often when using computer based performance assessments	B
Computer based performance assessments are often frustrating	C
I need additional instructions to use computer based performance assessments	D
Using computer based performance assessments require a lot of mental effort	E
I find it easy to recover from errors in computer based performance assessments	F
Using computer based performance assessments are rigid and inflexible to interact with	G
I find it easy to get computer based performance assessments to do what I want it to do	H
The computer based performance assessments often acts in unexpected ways	I
I find it cumbersome to use computer based performance assessments	J
It is easy to remember how to perform tasks using computer based performance assessments	K
Computer based performance assessments can provide helpful guidance in performing tasks	L
Overall, I find computer based performance assessments easy to use	M

APPENDIX B

LIST OF ACRONYMS

AI……………………………………………………………………..…...…Artificial Intelligence
CEX………………………………………………………………..Clinical Evaluation Exercise
DARPA……………………………….........Defense Advanced Research Project Agency
ECA…………………………………………………………...Embodied Conversational Agent
HCDCM……………………...…..Human-Centered Distributed Conversational Modeling
HOLOMER………………………...HOLO-graphic M-edical E-lectronic R-epresentation
IITSEC………Interservice/Interindustry Training, Simulation, and Education Conference
IRB……………………………………………………..……………Institutional Review Board
IPS………………………………………………..…………………..Interpersonal Simulator
Cex……………………………………………..……………………Clinical Evaluation Exercise
METI Lab……………………………………..Mixed Emerging Technology Integration Lab
NEX… ……………………...………………………………...Neurology Evaluation Exercise
NLP……………………………………………………………....…Natural Language Processing
PANAS……………………………………...…Positive and Negative Affects Schedule
OSCE………………………………………………Observed Structured and Clinical Evaluations
RFI……………………………………………………………….....……Request for Information
RITE…………………………………………Residency In-service Training Examination
SOAP…………………………………...……...Subjective, Objective, Assessment, and Plan
SME……………………………………...……………………………..Subject Matter Expert
SP…………………………………...………………………………………Standardized Patient
TED………………………………...………………….Technology Entertainment Design
UI…………………………………..…………………………………….....Urinary Incontinence
VERG…………………………..……………………………Virtual Environments Research Group
VH……………………………..………………………………………………......Virtual Human
VMS……………………...………………………………………………...Virtual Medical Student
V-people………………..……………………………………………………......Virtual People
VPF………………………………..……………………………………..…Virtual People Factory
WB………………………………..……………………………………………..…Web Based
3-D……………………………..………………………………………………Three Dimensional

APPENDIX C
CASE STUDIES

COMPUTER BASED VS TRADITIONAL TRAINING

The standardized patient program at USC allows the patient to train to simulate the signs and symptoms of actual patients. Some good candidates for these are people who have stable, abnormal physical findings. The students that are chosen are able to successfully reenact a scenario the same time, every time. This provides standardization in performance (Standardized, 2009).

SPs don't use this method at the moment as this is normally used for the training of medical students. SPs were used in a study that lasted over the span of two years. This SP curriculum was combined with two methods. This program was broken out into a computer based and traditional treatment in training. Post-test counseling was the main training objective (Konkle, 2002). There were approximately 500 people or more of these individuals who were located in rural areas. These geographic areas provided positive results. The awareness and capability to perform in clinical practice was strengthened as a result. Furthermore, there is a strengthened sense of being able to mitigate and detect risks for the subjects.

The electronic delivery of training content for medicine is becoming a growing trend. Some of these computer based training tools have other features such as allowing a student to go back and remediate themselves when questions were answered incorrectly. However, there has not been significant research that discovers how these self-delivered educational programs provide a benefit in learning transfer for standardized patients (Errichetti,

2006). This study is essential in providing a comparison between the traditional techniques of acting out a scenario and being given training as opposed to a computer based training method. The comparison also shows if there is any value or new discoveries that can be found when using the computer based training. To analyze this data, the groups were split up among the two modalities and their abilities in reenacting the cases were based on how they were trained and evaluated (Errichetti, 2006). This group consisted of forty medical students. These medical students were required to participate in a clinical skills assessment where they had to be involved in 5 different stations that had different requirements. Some of the subjects had a computer trained SP while others had an SP that was trained by an instructor. This interaction was recorded and archived for further analysis, debrief, and education. Findings of the data showed that there is a larger and better accuracy of the standardized patient skills that were part of the computer-based trained group. In addition, although the traditionally trained SPs were more realistically performed, the metrics displayed that they were considered less dependable than the computer trained group. This study supports that the development of an integrated training process that is created on a computer based training medium can allow medical students to work with standardized patients who are not only more dependable, but prepared. Educational programs that are delivered electronically to students can provide a benefit in learning concepts in the medical realm (Errichetti, 2006). With this information, we can realize another dimension can be introduced to standardize patient training. The integration of these dimensions provides a solution that is more powerful than what currently exists. Below is a comparison of the different modalities from a literature study.

Table 11: SP Training Modality Comparison Matrix

	Reading a Scenario	Training Model	Human Training/ Mentorship	Computer Based Training	Integrated Training	Avatars	Video	Audio Recording	Web-based	Didactic	Virtual People Factory	Roleplay Trainer	Inter-personal Simulator	Experiential Learning	ECAs	Team Based ECA	HCDCM
Churchill, 1999																	
Conkey, 2010																	
Errichetti, 2006																	
Furman, 2008																	
Halan, 2010																	
Kobak, 2006																	
Kolb, 2001, 1984																	
Konkle, 2002																	
Kurzwell, 2003																	
Lee, 2006																	
Lester, 1997																	
May, 2008																	
Palathinkal, 2010																	
Poggl, 1991																	
Tamblyn, 2010																	
Turner, 2006																	
Rickel, 1999																	
Rossen, 2010																	

CROSSOVER STUDY BETWEEN STANDARDIZED PATIENT AND WEB BASED TRAINING

Another study is conducted as a crossover study to compare results of web based training and traditional standardized patient training. Within the last 10 years, there have been larger needs for standardized patient training (Turner, 2006). The United States greatly utilizes these approaches to get medical students, physicians, and healthcare advocates the experience they need. The SP provides a very valuable tool in clinical skills for physicians (Turner, 2006). There is a cost savings aspect to this as a standardized patient encounter is a more economical choice when compared to the faculty-led pursuits.

The article written by Turner supports that the methods of teaching clinical reasoning continues to evolve. Although there are still good approaches, there are still opportunities to improve the process (Turner, 2006). When comparing Standardized Patient (SP) training to Web-based (WB) training, SP training is proven to be more effective than lectures, and Web-based training is a little less clear in its consistency. One study showed WB training to be beneficial for some physical examination skills (Turner, 2006). However, there were four other tests that showed no correlation to the modality of training (Tuner, 2006). However, some things that have been considered an advantage to using the web-based training tool was being able to train several times, a shorter learning curve, and data that updates often (Turner, 2006). In addition, a learning management system could be added to provide for a better ease of use in customizability in content. The clinical portion of the Step 2 CS exam has caused more of a need in standardization. However, as previously stated, there have not been too many studies which compare the results from training two methodologies of training (Turner, 2006).

A study is performed at the University of Nevada School Of Medicine. It consists of fifty-four students in their second year at the college of medicine. A randomized computer number generator is used to have the groups split into two sections. These two groups are known as "Cohorts 1 and 2". Cohort 1 involved the subjects to first go through some WB instruction and then have SP instruction (Turner, 2006). The second cohort was called "Cohort 2", which first had SP instruction. This Cohort was later followed by WB instruction (Turner, 2006). Both tracks of training consisted of two sequential learning modules. The first session was a case consistent of abdominal pain, and then the case to later follow was involving a headache (Turner, 2006).

The WB case had a software package that was developed called: DxR Clinician® (DxR Development Group, Carbondale, IL), which was part of the modality. Students would begin their exercise by logging into a computer where the program would begin the cases with either the abdominal pain or headache scenario (Turner, 2006). An administrator was given authority to facilitate access of training material restricted to only randomize subjects during a 45 minute period of time.

The SP learning tasks were specific to particular medical scenarios (Turner, 2006). After each learning session, a medical educator would provide five minutes of feedback which was delivered via vocal feedback (Turner, 2006). The focus was to make both modalities as comparable as possible (Turner, 2006). The SP actors also were expected to be trained in a consistent way with reliability (Turner, 2006).

Checklists are used by standardized patients for rating medical students on their performance. For the SP cases, a physical checklist is used by faculty and physicians, while the WB modality utilized a computer. Both are good options, but this study shows which a better application is. Four days afterwards, both assessments have information to debrief the experience. This debrief includes an assessment plan, the checklists, and a breakdown of the differences in diagnosis. After four weeks, both cohorts are required to be involved in a follow-up exam. These results show if there is a learning transfer for the concepts of clinical reasoning. The exam takes 20 minutes to complete, and during this time, faculty members are involved in observing and evaluating the performance. The graded scores are based on blinded allocation of the cohorts (Turner, 2006). A Cronbach's alpha is used to analyze SOAP (subjective, objective, assessment, and plan) notes and checklists. The alpha is utilized often to verify that the test scores are within a favorable range (Chronbach, 2009). When each teaching session is completed, the students complete a text survey on the experience (Turner, 2006). The data is captured with the use of a Likert-Scale survey. The range is from a number 1 which is annotated as a strongly disagree to a number five which resembles a strongly agree (Turner, 2006). Costs are accounted for with regards to faculty and technical support costs which were approximately fifty dollars an hour (Turner, 2006). Furthermore, there are ongoing costs depending on the length of the studies and follow-on advancements which conclude to approximately $45 per an SP case and $30 for the WB case formats (Turner, 2006). So the upfront costs are cheaper for the SP, but the ongoing costs are cheaper when heading to a WB platform. The statement can be made that some types of web-based training incur more additional upfront costs for development and deployment; but provides cheaper ongoing costs.

When analyzing the statistics, the tests are utilized for the purpose of analyzing SOAP note and checklist scores. Statistical significance is demonstrated if the probabilities of values are less than .05. As a result, a Cronbach's alpha of .69 is provided and a .68 for the SOAP note is given. Both cohorts have similar consenting rates, and unfortunately do not show statistical significance. The p value is .06, which is a derivative of 75% of the sample being nonconsenters, and only 47% being consenters. What can be concluded from this is that learning with both WB and SP methods can provide grades that are within a close range of diagnosis for abdominal pain and headache SOAP notes. When considering the WB modality, there was a better grade when it came to testing of the abdominal pain but not when analyzing the headache.

MEDICAL STUDENT PERFORMANCE WITH RICH MEDIA

Various cases can show approaches that lead to results in performance and statistics. This case compares and analyzes the modality of implementing a rich media web module for medical training. It is not directly used for standardized patient training for the Step 2 CS exam. However, this rich media module is actually used for better awareness for dangerous drinking (Lee, 2006). A standardized patient is used in comparison with the traditional lecture (Lee, 2006). There was a web based training session that was used to deliver pre and post tests, Flash©, and text didactics (Lee, 2006). There were videos on two alcohol cases. Both of these videos were comparisons of a beginner and experienced examiner (Lee, 2006). A primary purpose of this training is also to enhance communication skills. There has not been an extensive amount if any of published studies on this topic (Lee, 2006). Along with these communication skills, students are taught various topics that are in relation to the subjects of public and behavioral areas. The different methods in training are inclusive of lectures, web modules, and course syllabi. These methods assist in preparing the students for faculty-facilitated seminars (Lee, 2006). The three current parts to the curriculum consist of a lecture, small group seminar, and an OSCE (observed structured and clinical evaluations case).

For the study, the first class of 2006-2007 medical students was chosen as a cohort. The sample of N=163 was assigned to participate in a web module which was paired with a one hour lecture. However, an interesting point to observe is that both the web-based training and the lecture were optional (Lee, 2006). Within 3-5 weeks, the two groups joined meetings with a patient that is involved in hazardous drinking; which later had an OSCE alcohol case (Lee, 1006). Demographic data was not collected as a result to restrictions of the NYUSOM IRB as the population did not have a significant amount of diversity.

The web based module that was preferred, was java-based. This was developed by the NYU Division of Educational Informatics faculty. This website can be accessed at the url: http://edinfo.med.nyu.edu/alcoholscreening/ (Lee, 2007). The login is the word: demo; and the password is: demo) (Lee, 2007). For the duration of the week, students were allowed to use an ID and password to login to the module where they would agree to submit their responses for the contribution of research. The pretest consisted of multiple choice questions that ranked answers based on a scale (Lee, 2007). This was used to get the learner accustomed to educational information along with understanding gaps in knowledge (Lee, 2007). The knowledge sections included safe drinking limits and also provided background information for two alcohol vignettes (Lee, 2007). In addition, there was a separate area which had an outline that decomposed the learning modules. A voice over provided the feature to have audio narration. This also keyed in on particular areas of interest. Many of these highlighted principles used the applications of Flash© animation and hyperlinks to external sources (Lee, 2007). This was a great cost savings application as it reduced the need for extraneous text which could be leveraged from other sources. Two video clips were used to illustrate teaching and training as part of the curriculum (Lee, 2007). One of the videos consisted was a male with pancreatitis who is attempting to stop drinking and the other video has a person of the opposite sex who fails to follow a reasonable amount of alcohol levels and later decreases the amount that is consumed (Lee, 2007). Later, an inexperienced student's interview was followed by a physician who was in the field for a long time which had expert examples of interview techniques (Lee, 2007). After each 1-3 minute clip, the learner responded by typing in an area to input the text. Afterwards, the responses to the learner responses were coupled with the responses of the teachers (Lee, 2007). When this was complete, there was a posttest which had the same pre-test items; comparisons of the answers, and finally a module feedback prompt (Lee, 2007). The time duration of this was approximately 45 minutes. The lecture had the same steps for the procedures (Lee, 2007). Afterwards, there were small group seminars (Lee, 2007). Three to five weeks after the web and lecture training, an OSCE using SPs with two cases was put in place (Lee, 2007). Female SPs were educated and trained on roleplaying a woman character that reduced the intake of alcohol and was later evaluated and assessed individually (Lee, 2007). The SPs did not know if they were either lectured or WB (Lee, 2007).

The study had a sample of 82 subjects which was compared to the sample of N=81 groups who studied a lecture. A similar amount of students signed up for the web–based in comparison to the lecture training. It was 82% to 72%.

There were reasonable results from this trial version of a web-based training module. This web-based training represented a great tool for intervention of hazardous drinking. It was a great training for clinical skills for medical students. A significant amount of the students chose to use the web-based training as opposed to the lecture version of instruction. 5% of the lectured students were defected to the web training as a result of course instructions (Lee, 1008). 6 out of the 75 had some technical difficulty when using the computer. Constructive criticism from the students allowed the maintenance of a list of processes that could be improved (Lee, 2008). This was especially significant when expressing that the students preferred the web based training in comparison to the lecture (Lee, 2008). The web based training results were just as good as the lecture based training (Lee, 2008). There were better assessments of a patient's hazardous drinking.

However, there are some things that can be improved with the system (Lee, 2008). Presenter bias may have happened as a result of web authors being involved in the training sessions (Lee, 2008). SPs were expected to have higher reliability, but they occasionally overestimated student performance (Lee, 2008). Finally, some of these results were not beneficial to the students but show that web based training can be analyzed to ensure applied measures for clinical skills (Lee, 2008). These applications should be justified for cost and effectiveness (Lee, 2009). In conclusion, this is another instance where web-based training provides a positive result for training and automated assessment. Web based training is chosen as a more preferred medium when compared to traditional lecture based training. Not only is it a preferred choice, but it is more convenient for students.

FINAL WORDS

This book is a fresh look into Standardized Patient education. The concepts of this book not only look into what futurists see as the future of healthcare, clinical skills education and surgery, but also provide in depth details on some experiences that SPs, medical students, educators, and physicians face. It is the medical students that depend on the quality of SPs to have a fair trial when taking board exams. In retrospect some things that were talked about were what SPs are, the issues, learning gaps, and needs that are required to improve SP education. Furthermore, the concept of virtual humans, embodied conversational agents, fundamentals of acting, clinical play, virtual humans, and future immersive technologies and simulation can get us to a better level of quality when educating these essential medical role players. Your interest in this topic is greatly appreciated, and hopefully your expertise will also provide an asset to the improvement of education in medicine.

REFERENCES

Adjoudani, A., and C. Benoit. 1996. On the integration of auditory and visual parameters in an HMM-based ASR. In D.G. Stork and M.E. Hennecke, eds., *Speechreading by humans and machines: Models, systems, and applications*, 461-472. Berlin: Springer-Verlang

Albright, H.D. Working up a Part. A Manual for the Beginning Actor. The Houghton Mifflin Company. The Riverside Press. Cambridge. 1959

Andre, E, and T. Rist. 1995. Generating coherent presentations employing textual and visual material. *Artificial Intelligence Review* 9(2-3):147-165. (Special issue on the Integration of Natural Language and Vision Processing.)

Association of Standardized Patient Educators. Retrieved on December 3rd, 2011. http://www.aspeducators.org

Azarbeyejani, A., C. Wren, and A. Pentland. 1996. Real time 3-D tracking of the human body. In Proceedings of IMAGE'COM 96 (Bordeaux, France), May

Badler, N., M. Palmer. And R. Bindiganavale. 1999. Animation control for real time virtual humans. Communications of the ACM 42(7):65-73.

Baker, Ann C, Jensen, Patricia J, & Kolb, David A. (2005). Conversation as Experiential Learning. Management Learning, 36(4), 411-427. Retrieved November 4, 2010, from ABI/INFORM Global. (Document ID: 944428841).

Ballenstedt, Brittany. Social Proof is the New Marketing. Techcrunch. Retrieved on November 29th, 2011 at http://techcrunch.com/2011/11/27/social-proof-why-people-like-to-follow-the-crowd/

Baker, A. C., Jensen, P. J. and Kolb, D. A. (1997) 1In Conversation: Transforming Experience into Learning'. Simulation and Gaming28(1): 6-12

Ball, G., Ling, D Kurlander, J Miller, D. Pugh, et al 1997. Lifelike computer characters: The persona project at Microsoft Research. In J.M. Bradshaw, ed., Software agents, 191-222. Menlo park, Calif: AAAI Press/The MIT Press.

Bavelas, J., N Chovil L, Coates, and L. Roe 1995. Interactive gestures. Dicourse processes 15:469-489

Beatty, G. W. 1981 Sequential temporal patterns of speech and gaze in dialogue. In T.A Sebeok and J Umiker-Sebeok, eds. Nonverbal communication, interaction, and gesture: Selections from Semiotica, 298-320. The Haugue: Mouton

Behrend, Tara S., Thompson, Lori Foster (2011). Similarity Effects in Online Training: Effects with Computerized Trainer Agents. Journal of Computers in Human Behavior. Volume 27, Issue 3. Elsevier Science Publishers B.V. Amsterdam, Netherlands.

Blog. Wikipedia Search. Retrieved on December, 8th, 2011

Bolan, CM. 2003 Incorporating the ***experiential learning*** theory into the instructional design of online courses. Nurse Educator 2003 Jan-Feb; Vol. 28 (1), pp. 10-4.

Bolt, R A 1980. Put-That-There: Voice and Gesture at the graphics interface. Computer Graphics 14 (3):262-270.

Bradley, C., Webb, T., Schmitz, C., Chipman, J., & Brasel, K. (2010). Structured teaching versus experiential learning of palliative care for surgical residents. *American Journal Of Surgery*, *200*(4), 542-547. Retrieved from MEDLINE database.

Bruner, Jerome S. (1983) Child's Talk: Learning to use language. New York: Norton.

Bruner, Jerome S. (1986) Play, Thought, and language. *Prospects, 16, 77-83.*

Bruner, Jerome S. (1990). *Acts of Meaning.* Cambridge, MA: Harvard University Press.

Cassell, Justine. (2000). Embodied Coversational Agents. MIT Press

Cassell, Justine . Research page. Retrieved on January 19th, 2012 at http://www.justinecassell.com/jc_research.htm

Coquelin, Constant. The Actor and His Art. Boston, Roberts, 1881 The Monograph which started a war of words

Chronbach's Alpha, *Wikipedia* retrieved on March 4, 2010 from http://en.wikipedia.org/wiki/Cronbach's_alpha

Cronbach, L. J. (1951). Coefficient alpha and the internal structure of tests. Psychometrika, 16(3), 297-334.

Churchill, E. F., L. Cook, P. Hodgson, S. Prevost, and J. W. Sullivan. 1999. Designing embodied conversational agent allies. A scenario based approach. FX Palo Alto Technical Report FXPAL-TR-99-023

Conkey, Curtis A. (2009). Video Based Soft Skills Training dissertation for Doctor of Philosophy in Modeling and Simulation in the College of Sciences at the University of Central Florida Orlando, Florida

Corty, Eric. (2006). Using and Interpreting Statistics: A practical text for the health, behavioral, and social sciences. Mosby; 1 Edition (September 25, 2006).

Davis, F.D.: Percieved usefulness, perceived ease of use, and user acceptance of information technology. MIS quarterly 13 (3), 319-340 (1989)

Dickerson, R., et al.: Evaluating a Script-Based Approach for Simulating Patient-Doctor Interaction. In: SCS 2005 International Conference on Human-Computer Interface Advances for Modeling and Simulation, pp. 79–84 (2005)

Diener, E., Larsen, R. J., Levine, S., & Emmons, R. A. (1985). Intensity and frequency: Dimensions underlying positive and negative affect. *Journal of Personality and Social Psychology, 48*, 1253-1265.

Dodson, Sarah, L. Body and Language. Intercultural Learning Through Drama. Understanding Drama Based Education. 2002

Doleman, John. The Art of Acting. Bonanza Books. Harper & Brothers New York. 1949

Duncan, S. 1974. Some signals and rules for taking speaking turns in conversations. In S. Weitz, ed., Nonverbal communication. New York: Oxford University Press

Errichetti A, Boulet JR. 2006 Oct;81(10 Suppl):S91-4. Comparing traditional and computer-based training methods for standardized patients. *Academic Medicine: Journal of the Association of American Medical Colleges.*

Faul, F., Erdfelder, E., Lang, A.-G., & Buchner, A. (2007). G*Power 3. A flexible statistical power analysis program for the social, behavioral, and biomedical sciences. *Behavior Research Methods, 39*, 175-191.

Feldman, M. (2008). *Controlling Our Emotion at Work: Implications for Interpersonal and Cognitive Task Performance in a Customer Service Simulation.* Unpublished Dissertation, University of Central Florida, Orlando, Florida.

First Aid for the USMLE Step 2 CS

Flanagan, Christine July 9, 2008. Meet a pioneer in surgical robotics and telemedicine: Dr. Richard Satava. Retrieved on January 15, 2012 at http://businessinnovationfactory.com/weblog/archives/2008/07/meet_a_pioneer.html

Foster, Noseworthy, Shah, Lind, Lok, Chuah, Rossen (2010). "Evaluation of Medical Student Interaction with a Bipolar Virtual Patient Scenario Written by a Peer Support Specialist – a Pilot Study". Poster. ADMSEP 2010, Jackson Hole, WY, June 17-19, 2010.

Foster, Londino, Noseworthy, Lind, Shah, Lok, Chuah, Rossen, "The Use of Interactive Virtual Patients in an Integrated Psychiatry-Neuroanatomy Course and a Psychiatry Clerkship". Plenary accepted to *ADMSEP 2010*, Jackson Hole, WY, June 17-19, 2010.

Funke, L., & Booth, J.E. (1961). Actors Talk About Acting. Random House: New York.

Furman GE. (2008). The role of standardized patient and trainer training in quality assurance for a high-stakes clinical skills examination. *Kaohsiung Journal of Medical Science.* 24(12):651-5.

Fussell, Holly E. , Lewy, Colleen S. and McFarland, Bentson H.(2009) 'Evaluating and Training Substance Abuse Counselors: A Pilot Study Assessing Standardized Patients as Authentic Clients', Substance Abuse, 30:1, 47 - 60

Halan, Shiva, Rossen, Brent, Cendan, Juan, Lok, Benjamin (2010). "High Score! – Motivation Strategies for User Participation in Virtual Human Development". Short Paper. *10th International Conference on Intelligent Virtual Agents (IVA)*, Philadelphia, Pennsylvania, Sept. 20-22, 2010.

Hall, Judith A. 2009. Jan 6th. Patient Education and Counseling. Observer Rated Rapport in interactions between medical students and standardized patients.

Heeter, C. (1992). Being there: the subjective experience of presence. *PRESENCE: Teleoperators and Virtual Environments, 1*(2), 262-271.

Holt, Chris. How to Become a Video Game Actor. Gamepro Retrieved on December 3rd 2011 at http://www.gamepro.com/article/features/222114/how-to-become-a-video-game-voice-actor/

Hooks, Ed., Acting for Animators: A complete guide to animators: A complete guide to performance animation, revised edition (Portsmouth, NHL Heinemann, 2003)

Ieronutti, L., & Chittaro, L. (2007). Employing virtual humans for education and training in X3D/VRML worlds. *Computers & Education, 49*(1), 93-109.oi:10.1016/j.compedu.2005.06.007.

Improv Encyclopedia. (2011). Boal, Augosto. Theater of the Oppressed. Retrieved on December 3rd, 2011 at http://improvencyclopedia.org/references//Theater_of_the_Oppressed.html.

Johnson, W. L., J. Rickel, R. Stiles, and A. Munro. (1998). Integrating pedagogical agents into virtual environments. *PRESENCE: Teleoperators and Virtual Environments, 7 (6):523-546.*

Johnsen, J., D. Beck, B. Lok. (2010). "The Impact of a Mixed Reality Display Configuration on User Behavior with a Virtual Human", *10th International Conference on Intelligent Virtual Agents (IVA 2010)*, Philadelphia, Pennsylvania, Sept. 20-22, 2010 – LNCS Proceedings.

Karlowicz, K. (2009). Evaluation of the Urinary Incontinence Scales to Measure Change After Experiential Learning: A Pilot Study. *Urologic Nursing, 29*(1), 40-46.

Retrieved from Health Source: Nursing/Academic Edition database.

Kobak, K., Engelhardt, N., & Lipsitz, J. (2006). Enriched rater training using Internet based technologies: A comparison to traditional rater training in a multi-site depression trial. Journal of Psychiatric Research, 40(3), 192199.doi:10.1016/j.jpsychires.2005.07.012.

Kolb, D. A. (1984). Experiential learning: experience as the source of learning and development: Prentice-Hall Englewood Cliffs, New Jersey.

Kolb, D. A., Boyatzis, R. E., & Mainemelis, C. (2001). Experiential Learning Theory: Previous Research and New Directions. Perspectives on Thinking, Learning, and Cognitive Styles.

Kolb D. University of Puget Sound Web site. Available at: http://www.ups.edu/aca/advman/mbdevl2.htm. Accessed March 24, 2003.

Kolb DA. Experiential Learning. Englewood Cliffs, NJ: Prentice-Hall; 1984;77–78,141

Konkle-Parker, D., Cramer, C., & Hamill, C. (2002). Standardized patient training: a modality for teaching interviewing skills. *Journal Of Continuing Education In Nursing, 33*(5), 225-230. Retrieved from MEDLINE database.

Kotranza, A., D. Lind, C. Pugh, and B. Lok, "Virtual Human + Tangible Interface = Mixed Reality Human. An Initial Exploration with a Virtual Breast Exam Patient" *IEEE Virtual Reality 2008*, March 8-12, Reno, NV, 99-106.

Krasnor and Pepler (1980). The study of children's play: Some suggested future directions. New Directions for Child Development, 9, 85-94.

Lagnado, Lucette. These Lagnado Take Dramatic Turns at the Hospital: To Help Train Doctors, Actors Get Gigs Playing Patients; Nabbing a Gout Role. The Wall Street Journal. Tuesday August 126th, 2011. Vol CCLVII No. 39

L. A. Schuh. Education Research: Bias and poor interrater reliability in evaluating the Neurology Clinical Skills Examination. *Neurology* 2009;73;904-908; originally published online Jul 15, 2009; DOI: 10.1212/WNL.0b013e3181b35212

Lee, J., Triola, M., Gillespie, C., Hanley, K., Zabar, S., Kalet, A., et al. (2008). Working with patients with alcohol problems: A controlled trial of the impact of a rich media web module on medical student performance. Journal of General Internal Medicine, 23(7), 1006-1009. doi:10.1007/s11606-008-0557-5

Lee, E-J., and C. Nass. 1998. Does the ethnicity of a computer agent matter? An experimental comparison of human-computer interaction and computer-mediated communication. In proceedings of the workshop on embedded Conversational Characters Conference (Lake Tahoe, Calif)

Lester, James C., Deictic and Emotive Communication in Animated Pedagogical Agents (2000). Embodied Conversational Agents. MIT Press

Lester et al., 1997 Lester, J. C., Converse, S. A., Kahler, S. E., Barlow, S. T., Stone, B. A., & Bhogal, R. S. (1997). The persona effect: affective impact of animated pedagogical agents. In *Proceedings of CHI '97.*

Mancini, Flavia, Longo, Mathew. 2011. Visual Distortion of Body Size Modulates Pain Perception. Psychological Science

Massaro, D. W., and M. M Cohen. 1977. Voice onset time and fundamental frequency as cues to the /zi/-/si/distinction. Perception and Psychphysics 22:373-382

May W. 2008. Training standardized patients for a high-stakes Clinical Performance Examination in the California Consortium for the Assessment of Clinical Competence. *Kaohsiung Journal of Medical Science* 24(12):640-5

McNaughton, Nancy. Effects of Portraying Psychologically and Emotionally Complex Standardized Patients. Teaching and Learning in Medicine. Volume 11, Issue 3, 1999.

Metcalf, David S. 2006 Keynote address video: Distance Learning 2006 at the University of Wiscon sin, Madison. Retrieved on February 4th 2012 at http://www.davidmetcalf.com/blog/2006/08/dr_david_metcalf_keynotes_dl06.html

Meier, U., R. Stiefelhagen, and J. Yang. (1997). Preprocessing of visual speech under real world conditions. In C. Benoit and R. Cambell, eds., Proceedings of the ESCA Workshop on Audio Visual Speech Processing, Cognitive and Computational

Approaches. (Rhodes, Greece), 113-116.

Mistry, Pranav. (2009). The Thrilling Potential of Sixth Sense Technology, TED lecture. http://www.ted.com/talks/pranav_mistry_the_thrilling_potential_of_sixthsense_technology.html. Retrieved on August 20, 2011.

Mott V.W. (2000). The development of professional expertise in the workplace. New directions for Adult and Continuing Education 86: 23-31.

Napier, Mark. Improvise. Scene from the Inside Out. Heinemann. 2004

Nass, C., and L. Mason. 1990. On the study of technology and task: A variable based approach. In J. Fulk and C. Stienfeld, eds., Organizations and communication technology, 46-67. Newbury park, Calif: Sage

NASA. 1993 CLIPS reference manual. Technical Report, Software Technology Branch, Lyndon B. Johnson Space Center

O'Connell, Vanessa. At GE, Robo-Lawyers. (2011) Oil and Gas Unit Tests Online Resolution to Control Costs. Wall Street Journal. Business Technology.

Optale, G., Urgesi, C., Busato, V., Marin, S., Piron, L., Priftis, K., et al. (2010). Controlling memory impairment in elderly adults using virtual reality memory training: a randomized controlled pilot study. *Neurorehabilitation And Neural Repair*, *24*(4), 348-357. Retrieved from MEDLINE database.

Pettit, H, and M. Beth. (2009). Research Plans and Joint Medical Simulation Technology (JMST) IPT briefing.

Phillips, R., & Bonsteel, S. (2010). The faculty and information specialist partnership: stimulating student interest and experiential learning. *Nurse Educator*, *35*(3), 136-138. Retrieved from MEDLINE database.

Plantec, Peter., Kurzweil, Ray. Virtual Humans: A build it yourself kit, complete with software and step-by-step instructions. 2003

Poggi, I. 1991. La communicazione. In R. Asquini and P. Lucisano, eds., L'Italiano nella scuola elementare. Aspetti linguisti. Florence: La Nuova Italia.

Privateer, P. M. (1999). Academic Technology and the Future of Higher Education: Strategic Paths Taken and Not Taken. *The Journal of Higher Education, 70(1), 60.*

Rickel, J. and W.L. Johnson 1999a. Animated agents for procedural training in virtual reality perceptionents for procedural training in virtual reality: perception, cognition, and motor control. Applied artificial intelligence 13: 343-382

Rossen, Brent, Cendan, Juan, Lok, Benjamin (2010). "Using Virtual Humans to Bootstrap the Creation of Other Virtual Humans". Short Paper. *10th International Conference on Intelligent Virtual Agents (IVA)*, Philadelphia, PA, Sept. 20-22, 2010.

Rossen, B., Lind, D.S., Lok, B (2009). Human-centered Distributed Conversational Modeling: Effi cient Modeling of Robust Virtual Human Conversations. In: Ruttkay, Z., Kipp, M., Nijholt, A., Vilhjálmsson, H.H. (eds.) IVA 2009. LNCS, vol. 5773, pp. 474–481. Springer, Heidelberg.

Rossen, B. SP Case link for interaction at http://vpf/cise.ufl.edu/VirtualPeopleFactory/public Overview.php?u=3535&script_id=424a on February 13, 2011.

Russ, Sandra W., Niec, Larissa N. (2011). Play in Clinical Practice: Evidence Based Approaches. The Guilford Press.

Sanders, G. A. and J. Scholtz. (1998). Measurement and evaluation in embodied conversational characters. *In Proceedings of the Workshop on Embodied Conversational Characters* (WECC 98) (Tahoe City, Calif.), 114-118, 85-86. (Pagination due to proceedings printing error.)

Sims, M Edward. Reusable, lifelike virtual humans for mentoring and role-playing. Computers & Education Volume 49, Issue 1, August 2007, Pages 75-92 Web3D Technologies in Learning, Education and Training

Sinek, Simon. How Great Leaders Inspire Action. Retreived on December 4th 2011 at http://www.youtube.com/watch?v=qp0HIF3SfI4

Sixth Sense Technology, Google Image Search

Smith S. (2008). MAN OF MANY FACES. *Men's Fitness* [serial online]. 24(10):88-93. Available from: Health Source - Consumer Edition, Ipswich, MA. Accessed December 4, 2011.

Smith, Roger. 2009. Game Technology in Medical Education. An inquiry into the Effectiveness of New Tools 1st ed.

Standardized Patient Program, MEDED. (2004) Retrieved July 22nd, 2009 from http://mededonline.usc.edu/sp.html

Stanislavinsky, Constantin. (1936). *An Actor Prepares.* Trans. Elizabeth Reynolds Hapgood. New York: Theater Arts, Inc.

Stanislavinsky, Constantin. (1949). *Building a Character.* Trans. Elizabeth Reynolds Hapgood. New York: Theater Arts, Inc.

Stanislavinsky, Constantin. My Life in Art. Trans. J. J Robbins. Boston: Little, Brown & Co., 1958

Stephan, W., and W.E. Beane. 1978. The effects of belief similarity and ethnicity on liking and attributions for performance. *Revista Interamericana de Psicologica 12:153-159*

Tamblyn, M Robin. (1991). Sources of unreliability and bias in standardized-patient rating. *Teaching and Learning in Medicine, Volume 3, Issue 2 1991 , pages 74 - 85*

Tamblyn, R.M., Klass, D.J., Schnabl, G.K., et al.: The accuracy of standardized patient presentation. Medical Education 25(2), 100–109 (2009)

Technological Singularity. Wikipedia. Retrieved on February 24, 2012 at http://en.wikipedia.org/wiki/Technological_singularity

Ti, L., Fun-Gee, C., Gee-Mei, T., Wah-Tze, T., Tan, J., Liang, S., et al. (2009). Experiential learning improves the learning and retention of endotracheal intubation. *Medical Education*, *43*(7), 654-660. doi:10.1111/j.1365-2923.2009.03399.x.

Turner, M., Simon, S., Facemyer, K., Newhall, L., & Veach, T. (2006). Web-based learning versus standardized patients for teaching clinical diagnosis: a randomized, controlled, cross over trial. *Teaching And Learning In Medicine*, *18*(3), 208-214. Retrieved from

MEDLINE database. http://ezproxy.lib.ucf.edu/login?URL=http://search.ebscohost.com/login.aspx?direct=true&db=cmedm&AN=16776607&site=ehost-live

US Army, (2010). A Request for Information. Three Dimensional and Holographic Display Systems Technology Roadmap and Current Markey Survey. Medical Simulation Applications.https://www.fbo.gov/index?s=opportunity&mode=form&id=3c8707e2c17d3ee4a5b84bfd70a2f311&tab=core&_cview=0

Virtual Soldier Project (2011). DARPA. Retrieved on February 24th, 2011 at http://www.virtualsoldier.us/holomer.htm

Vygotsky, Lev S. (1996). Play and its role in the mental development of the child. Societ Psychology, 12 62-76

Vygotsky, Lev S. (1978). Mind in Society: The development of higher psychological processes. Eds. M. Cole, V. John-Steiner, S. Scribner, & E. Souberman Eds. Campbridge, MA: Harvard Uni versity Press.

Wagner, Betty Jane. (2002). Body and Language. Intercultural Learning Through Drama. Under standing Drama Based Education.

Wallace, Peggy. (2007). Coaching Standardized Patients: For Use in the Assessment of Clinical Competence. New York, Springer Publishing Company

Wessel, J., Williams, R., Finch, E., et al. (2003). Reliability and validity of an objective structured clinical examination for physical therapy students. Journal of Allied Health 32(4), 266–269.

Wikipedia Search on Trending. Retrieved on December 3rd http://en.wikipedia.org/wiki/Trending_topic

Wilks, Yorick, and Catizone, Roberta. (2010). Computer Speech and Language 25: A prototype for a conversational companion for reminiscing about images. University of Sheffield, Computer Science Department,

Wilks, Yorick, (ed.). (2010). Close Engagements with Artificial Companions: Key social, psychological, ethical and design issues. xxii, 315 pp. (pp. 11–20)

Wirth, Jeff. Interactive Acting: Acting, Improvisation, and Interacting for Audience Participatory Theatre. 1994.

Woodward, J., Carnine, D., & Gersten, R. (1988). Teaching Problem Solving Through Computer Simulations. American Educational Research Journal, 25(1), 72-86.

Wordnet Homepage. Available at: wordnetweb.princeton.edu/perl/webwn. Retrieved on December 18, 2010.

www.facebook.com

www.Twitter.com

www.ingramcontent.com/pod-product-compliance
Lightning Source LLC
Chambersburg PA
CBHW081542220326
41598CB00036B/6529